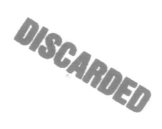
Male Infertility Guide for Couples

Male Infertility Guide
for Couples

**A Male Fertility Expert's "10 Week Man Plan"
to Maximize Fertility By Managing Low Sperm Counts,
Unexplained Infertility, and Recurrent IVF Failure**

Shane Russell, MD, MPH

Male Fertility Press, LLC

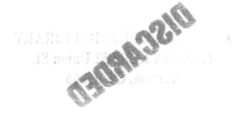

www.10weekmanplan.com

Disclaimer: The following information represents general male infertility management guidelines based upon the existing medical literature. Clinical decisions made for individual patients remain the responsibility of the clinician using their basic medical training and based upon the specific clinical situation.

ISBN-13: 978-0-9863532-2-2
Print Edition

Credits
Editor: Sue Warga
Formatting: Paul Salvette
Cover: SelfPubBookCovers.com/SilverhorseInk

This book is dedicated to Dr. Bob Brannigan, my mentor and friend, who introduced me to the fascinating world of male fertility and continues to serve as an inspiration on how to provide expert and compassionate care to couples going through an extremely stressful time in their lives.

Contents

Introduction

Infertility is a surprisingly common problem, affecting an estimated seven million couples in the United States. Given that it's such a widespread medical issue, one would expect to hear it talked about more often in the community. However, male infertility remains one of those topics that couples often keep to themselves, sometimes not even discussing it with their closest friends and relatives. Men are often particularly averse to talking about their own fertility problems (such as a low sperm count), as many feel shame and embarrassment that they are having difficulty fulfilling their reproductive contribution. The general lack of openness regarding male infertility can worsen the situation by making these men feel that they are one of only a very small number of men who suffer from these issues. The reality could hardly be further from the truth.

In the United States, approximately 15–20 percent of couples experience problems conceiving a child, and in 50 percent of these couples, male-factor fertility problems contribute to some extent to the inability to conceive. That adds up to *millions* of men, from all walks of life, experiencing fertility issues every year. The good news is that effective treatments exist for many of the most common causes of male-factor fertility problems. With the proper evaluation and treatment, the majority of couples with male fertility problems have the ability to conceive children who are biologically related to both parents.

Overcoming Roadblocks on the Path to Pregnancy

If treating male-factor infertility were universally easy, then this book would not be necessary. As with many aspects of life, worthwhile accomplishments often require a commitment of time and effort. In couples with fertility problems, both partners must be committed to making the changes needed to improve their chances of success. For men, who typically have been trying for years *not* to get anyone pregnant, this change of mind-set can sometimes be challenging.

Often, a major obstacle to managing male-factor fertility problems is successfully identifying a medical care provider who can offer competent assistance. Despite the large numbers of men who have trouble conceiving with their partner, the science and art of managing male infertility has remained largely neglected by the general medical community. The vast majority of primary care physicians have not been trained in even the basic principles of male fertility evaluation. Primary care doctors typically refer men with abnormal semen analyses to general urologists, who are supposed to be the "experts" in male fertility. Unfortunately, general urology training focuses primarily on treating problems such as kidney stones, enlarged prostates, bladder infections, incontinence, and cancer. Male infertility remains a relatively obscure field in most urology training programs, with very little formal fertility-related education being provided to urology residents during their training. To illustrate this point, a 2014 study published the findings of a survey of general urologists asking them how they manage male fertility problems. A full quarter of the surveyed general urologists reported giving men testosterone to treat fertility problems, despite the clearly established fact that giving a man testosterone causes sperm counts to dramatically *decrease*. This surprising lack of knowledge of even basic male fertility management guidelines underscores the poor state of general urologic training in caring for men with fertility problems.

Each year, a small number of urologists who have finished their general urology residency training decide to devote extra time to becoming experts in male fertility management by completing an additional one to two years of fellowship training in andrology, which is the branch of medicine concerned with disease affecting men, and particularly those affecting the male reproductive system. Unfortunately, the number of urologists who choose to become male fertility experts is quite small, with only eight fellowship training programs in the entire country, most of which produce just one graduate a year. In contrast, there are forty-three fellowship training programs in the United States to train female fertility specialists. This small number of fellowship-trained male fertility experts cannot possibly provide care to the three and a half million infertile couples in the United States who have male-factor problems. Most couples with male fertility issues must therefore rely upon a primary care physician or a general urologist for guidance. Faced with unsatisfying answers from their health care providers, couples often turn to the Internet, which, unfortunately, is filled with misinformation, half-truths, and conflicting recommendations. It is no wonder that so many infertile couples feel frustrated and hopeless.

The failure of basic medical training to provide education on male fertility problems, along with a general clinical emphasis on the female side of fertility, means that too often male infertility is overlooked and undertreated. The goal of this book is to start to change this view, and to provide the 50 percent of infertile couples who have male-factor problems with the tools to help navigate a course to a successful pregnancy.

The Purpose of This Book

The 10 Week Man Plan describes and explains the latest recommendations for evaluation and treatment of male-factor infertility.

If you are not working with a fellowship-trained expert in male fertility, this book can provide you with the basic knowledge necessary to make sure that the care you are receiving follows the basic guidelines of good male fertility medical care. If you are working with a male fertility specialist, then this book can help bring you up to speed on the basic language and general structure of male infertility management, thereby preparing you to have meaningful conversations with your physician and get the most out of your office consultations. Infertility problems can be complex, and you have only a limited amount of time with your doctor at each visit. A good baseline understanding of the factors that may be involved in male infertility can make visits to your doctor more effective and efficient, help you focus on the most important questions you want to get answered, and allow you to improve semen production as quickly as possible.

Having children is one of life's most basic impulses, and raising a family is generally considered to be one of the most rewarding (and, at times, challenging) pursuits that any person can choose to undertake. This book has been designed to give every couple suffering from male-factor problems the resources they might need to maximize their chances of fulfilling their fertility goals.

1

A Brief Overview of Normal Male Fertility

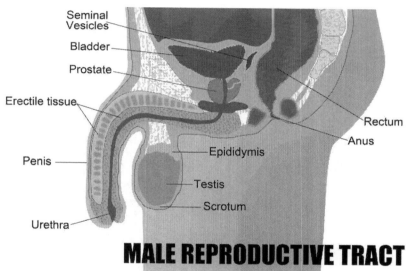

Seminal Vesicles

Bladder

Prostate

Erectile tissue

Rectum

Anus

Epididymis

Penis

Testis

Scrotum

Urethra

MALE REPRODUCTIVE TRACT

The 10 Week Man Plan is a guide for couples with either known male-factor infertility problems or unexplained infertility problems. The goal of the plan is to maximize each man's fertility potential to the greatest extent possible. In order to do this, it is helpful to understand how the fertility process works in couples who do not have trouble conceiving.

Normal Pregnancy Rates

When couples with no known infertility issues start trying to have a baby, their odds of achieving a pregnancy are about 15–25 percent each month. About 50–75 percent of these couples will have successfully established a pregnancy within six months, and 90 percent will have done so within one year. After a year of unsuccessful trying, however, a couple's chances of naturally establishing a pregnancy will have dropped to approximately 3–5 percent each month.

Normal Sperm Production

Sperm production is initiated and maintained by the male hormonal system. The pituitary gland, which sits at the base of the brain, is the hormonal "control center" of the body. Cells within the front part of the pituitary gland produce two very important hormones, follicle-stimulating hormone (FSH) and luteinizing hormone (LH). FSH induces the spermatogenic cells within the testicles to make sperm, while LH signals the Leydig cells within the testicles to make testosterone.

FSH and LH play complementary roles in normal sperm production. Without FSH, the spermatogenic cells would not make sperm. However, sperm production requires high testosterone levels within the testicles; hence the importance of LH stimulation to drive increased testosterone production.

Normal Sperm Maturation

Unlike women, who are born with all the eggs they will ever have, after puberty men continuously make new sperm. The sperm development process takes approximately ten weeks, as sperm precursor cells slowly transform into fully mature sperm. During this maturation process, the sperm leave the testicle and enter into the epididymis, a structure that wraps around the side of the testicle. When sperm leave the epididymis and enter into the long tube called the vas deferens, they are fully mature and ready to swim. Large numbers of sperm are concentrated within the vas deferens in preparation for future ejaculation.

Normal Male Sexual Function

The bulbourethral glands (also called Cowper's glands) are a pair of small glands that sit beneath the urethra near the prostate. During sexual intercourse, the bulbourethral glands produce a small amount of clear fluid (called pre-ejaculate) that lubricates the urethra and neutralizes the acidity of any residual urine left behind from the last urination. When ejaculation occurs, the vas deferens rhythmically contracts, forcing the sperm to flow into the ejaculatory ducts. Within the ejaculatory ducts, the sperm pick up fluid from the seminal vesicles, which then joins fluid from the prostate gland as it enters the urethra. Strong contractions of the surrounding muscles then force the sperm out of the urethra, through the tip of the penis, and into the woman's vagina.

Normal Conception

Following ejaculation, sperm are deposited near the woman's cervix, which is a structure at the top of the vagina leading into the uterus. The part of the ejaculate fluid that was produced by the seminal vesicles causes the semen to coagulate (stick together), and this helps to protect the sperm from the harsh, acidic environment of the vagina. The prostate fluid contains enzymes that gradually release the sperm from the coagulated mass of the rest of the ejaculated fluid, thereby allowing the sperm to enter the woman's cervix. Hormonal changes in women around the time of ovulation (when a mature egg is released from the ovary) cause the cervix to be more receptive to allowing sperm to pass into the uterus. The sperm then swim up the uterus into the fallopian tubes in search of an egg. During this process, the vast majority of the sperm will die. Only a small number of the fittest, best-swimming sperm actually make it up the fallopian tubes to the area where fertilization can occur. If the timing is right, these sperm will meet up with an egg that has been released from the woman's ovary. A single sperm will penetrate the egg, causing a chemical reaction within the egg that excludes any other sperm from entering as well. The miracle of fertilization and embryo development then ensues, with the embryo traveling down the rest of the fallopian tube and implanting within the wall of the uterus, the lining of which has thickened under hormonal influence to grow and provide the rich blood supply necessary to sustain a growing embryo.

Conception is a fascinating and complex process. Although it takes place within the female reproductive tract, the male contribution obviously plays a vital role and contributes half of the DNA of the future baby. With all of the myriad steps and mechanisms necessary for normal conception, it is amazing that the process proceeds normally in the majority of couples. There are many steps along the way, though, where problems can present themselves, and overcoming these obstacles to fertility on the male side is the focus of this book.

2

The 10 Week Man Plan
Where to Start

This book is intended to be useful for couples in all stages of the fertility process, whether they are just getting started or have been trying to conceive for many years.

How to Use This Book

The 10 Week Man Plan is not designed to be read straight through from start to finish. A wide range of potential problems can affect male fertility, and it can be frustrating and unhelpful for couples to have to wade through information on topics unrelated to their particular situation. This book has therefore been organized in a way that helps identify the topics that may be pertinent to you, and to guide you to those sections that are most relevant to your situation.

This book is also not a comprehensive review of all of the scientific studies that underpin the current recommendations for managing male infertility problems. There are several good technical textbooks that offer an overview of the basic scientific research and studies that underlie the practice guidelines for male fertility; see Appendix B for a list if you're interested in that level of detail. The goal of this book is to provide a set of basic guidelines and principles that are easy to understand and useful on a day-to-day basis for couples who do not have formal medical training.

As you go through the book, keep in mind that the recommendations provided here are general guidelines for a typical man. Health-related interventions and medication dosages listed are those generally used in most men, but these may need to be modified depending on each man's individual medical history, health status, and physical characteristics.

Finally, this is not intended to be a do-it-yourself guide. Working with a licensed and qualified medical care provider is mandatory for safe and effective management of male-factor fertility problems. The human body is a very complex system, and any interventions related to male fertility should be supervised by a trained medical professional. From a practical standpoint, most medical testing and prescription medications also need a signed order from a physician, physician assistant, or nurse practitioner.

If you have access to a fellowship-trained expert on male fertility in your area, it would definitely be in your best interest to work with that person. This specialist may not agree with every recommendation made in this book, and that is to be expected—if you spend any time with a group of specialists in any medical field, you'll quickly find that they disagree on many things. I have tried to point out common controversies among male infertility specialists and provide both sides of the basic arguments, to help facilitate further discussions on these topics with your physician. Appendix A offers some tips for finding a male infertility specialist in your region. If you do not have access to a fellowship-trained specialist, this book can help you to determine if the general urologist you are working with is using the latest management guidelines.

Since 50 percent of infertility is in some way related to male-factor issues, *all* male partners in couples with infertility problems should have a semen analysis done. This book explains how to arrange for accurate semen testing, interpret the results of the tests, and review the options if any abnormalities are discovered. It also provides you with sample forms for testing, the diagnostic codes that can be used, and general costs for the different tests if they are not covered by insurance. Diagnostic codes are number codes assigned to tests ordered by medical professionals; the codes are used by insurance companies for billing and to determine if coverage is available. The current coding system, called the ICD-9, is set to change to the new ICD-10 coding system on October 1, 2015 (unless the federal government decides to postpone this deadline). Both the ICD-9 and ICD-10 diagnostic codes have been included in this book.

Male Fertility and General Health Problems

Beyond the fact that the majority of male fertility problems are reversible, there are other reasons to evaluate men with problems such as a low sperm count or poor sperm quality. Some potentially significant health problems can be associated with decreases in male fertility potential. Rates of testicular cancer are three to thirty times higher in infertile males than in fertile males, and genetic abnormalities are thirty to a hundred times more common in this population. Overall, between 1 and 6 percent of men who undergo male fertility evaluations uncover some form of potentially serious underlying medical problem, such as prostate cancer, diabetes mellitus, hypothyroidism, or a brain tumor. If couples are sent straight to treatment from the female side (such as insemination procedures or in vitro fertilization) without evaluating the man, potentially serious medical problems could be missed.

A Note to My Medical Colleagues and Industry Representatives

As everyone is well aware, medicine is a combination of both art and science, and it is in a constant state of development and change. The content of this book is the product of ten years of clinical experience and a thorough review of the existing medical literature. Despite this, there will always be differences of opinion about how to handle certain clinical situations. I wholeheartedly welcome input from my colleagues for future editions of this book. I also encourage the pharmaceutical and medical device industry to provide feedback on new products and updated product information in order to keep future book editions as accurate as possible. Please feel free to contact me at 10weekmanplan@gmail.com.

Why Does the Plan Take Ten Weeks?

The 10 Week Man Plan presents a program designed to optimize the environment for sperm production by identifying and correcting any reversible male-factor issues that are present.

As Chapter 1 describes, the formation of mature sperm is a very complex physiologic process that takes place in a man's body over a ten-week period of time (called a spermatogenic cycle). A large number of factors play a role in determining the number and quality of sperm that are being produced. Some of these, such as genetic influences, are not under the man's control. However, a large number of factors that influence sperm production can potentially be modified and optimized. These potentially modifiable factors include:

Hormone levels

Lifestyle choices

Medications

Infections/inflammation

Job-related factors

Varicoceles

Erectile/ejaculatory problems

The 10 Week Man Plan is a comprehensive evaluation of all of these modifiable factors, with the goal of trying to maximize each man's own fertility potential effectively and efficiently.

Most of the women in couples who are reading this book want to be pregnant as soon as possible. For many, the process of trying to become a parent has been going on for many months already, and ten more weeks can seem like an eternity. However, the plan's timeline is a direct product of every man's basic physiology. It takes ten weeks for a sperm precursor cell from the testicles to transform into a mature sperm within the vas deferens that is ready to swim to and fertilize a woman's egg. Any positive or negative factors or events that occur during this ten-week period can impact the number and quality of sperm that are being produced during that spermatogenic cycle.

For example, if a man spends time in a hot tub, this can have a negative impact on all of the sperm that are currently in his body. It will then take about ten weeks for these potentially damaged sperm to clear the body and be replaced by an entirely new batch of sperm produced after the exposure to the hot tub.

Along the same lines, any positive changes that are made (such as quitting smoking, improved hormone levels, etc.) generally take around ten weeks to be fully reflected in the number and quality of sperm. The reason for this is that it takes this long for 100 percent of the sperm in the body to have been produced in the improved environment.

The length of the spermatogenic cycle therefore dictates the timeline of the 10 Week Man Plan. As you'll see, the basic structure of the plan is to improve the environment for sperm production as much as possible and then repeat fertility testing in ten weeks to reevaluate sperm quality. Of course, every couple's clinical situation is different, and specific circumstances may lead to modification of their individual plan's timeline.

For example, if a woman is forty-two years old, then waiting a full ten weeks to do a repeat semen analysis may not be in the couple's best interests—it might be a good idea to repeat the analysis sooner. On the other hand, some men require two spermatogenic cycles (twenty weeks) to see the full improvement in semen parameters following positive interventions. The human body is a complex system, and no two men (as well as no two couples) are exactly the same, so the ability to be flexible and modify the plan as the situation requires is important. For most men, however, a plan timeline that is ten weeks in length is ideal.

After all reversible male factor issues have been addressed and modified for ten weeks, most men can assume that their semen parameters have been optimized as much as possible (although some may continue to improve further with time). A key point in male fertility management is that all positive changes (lifestyle, hormonal, and so on) *should be continued until the woman is pregnant and through her first trimester*. If a man stops his interventions after the ten weeks are over, then the fertility improvements can be lost. And the chance of a woman losing a pregnancy substantially decreases after she has entered her second trimester, so it is generally recommended that men stay on the plan at least until the first trimester of pregnancy has passed (assuming everything is going fine with the pregnancy).

Where to Start

Whether you're just getting started in your efforts to conceive or you've been working on fertility issues for a while, *The 10 Week Man Plan* can help.

The first step is deciding which of seven basic scenarios you fall into. These scenarios include:

1. Just getting started (no male fertility testing yet)
2. Abnormal semen analysis findings
3. Normal semen analysis but still unable to conceive
4. Unable to successfully provide a specimen for semen analysis
5. Recurrent pregnancy loss
6. Recurrent IVF failure
7. Previous vasectomy

Each of these scenarios corresponds to a section below. These sections will guide you to the appropriate diagnostic and therapeutic pathways of the plan.

Just Getting Started

When should a couple who would like to have children undergo fertility testing? There are no strict guidelines here, as a couple's preferences play an important role in deciding when and if testing should be performed. However, general guidelines have been developed to give couples an idea of when fertility testing is typically initiated. These guidelines recommend that testing should be considered after:

- One year of unprotected intercourse without pregnancy if the woman is under thirty-five years of age and the man is under forty, *or*
- Six months of unprotected intercourse without pregnancy if the woman is thirty-five or older or the man is forty or older

Immediate testing can be considered in men with a known history of significant fertility risk factors, such as previous chemotherapy or radiation therapy, undescended testicles at birth, a personal history of testicular cancer, hormonal or genetic problems, or a history of anabolic steroid use.

As mentioned earlier, these are general guidelines that do not have to be followed exactly. Some young couples choose to wait a few years before testing, while others decide to undergo basic fertility testing prior to even starting trying to conceive, just to make sure that there is likely not going to be a problem. If this helps decrease stress and assist in their future planning, that's fine.

Since male-factor issues impact approximately 50 percent of couples who are having trouble conceiving, it is strongly recommended that both the male and female partners in a couple have basic fertility testing as part of an initial evaluation. From the male side, *two semen analyses performed at least ten weeks apart* is recommended for initial testing.

If you and your partner are just getting started with trying to conceive, begin with Chapter 3, which will review recommendations for getting a semen analysis performed the correct way and discuss interpretation of the results.

Abnormal Semen Analysis Findings

Many couples have already had semen testing performed, ordered either by their primary care physician, local urologist, or the woman's gynecologist. However, an accurate fertility picture cannot be obtained with just one semen analysis; I recommend men get *at least two analyses spaced at least ten weeks apart*. If a couple has had only one semen analysis (or two that were performed less than ten weeks apart, it's a good idea to get at least one more. This second test can be performed after completing the 10 Week Man Plan in order to see what effect an optimized environment for sperm production has had on the semen.

If you've already had one semen analysis, start with Chapter 3, to make sure that the testing was performed properly and to review the interpretation of the results before embarking on the 10 Week Man Plan.

Normal Semen Analysis but Still Unable to Conceive

Sometimes a couple who has been trying to conceive for at least a year end up having completely normal fertility test results from both the male and female sides. Some of this inability to conceive may be due to pure chance (that is, bad luck) and simply trying longer will eventually result in success. Other times there may be hidden factors that are not uncovered by routine semen analysis. Certainly there are physiologic aspects of male fertility that have not been discovered yet by scientific research and so cannot be currently tested for.

If no significant abnormalities are discovered after two normal semen analyses, and if fertility testing for the woman has produced normal results, a couple has several options:

- *Optimize the environment for sperm production with the 10 Week Man Plan.* Even if the results of the semen analysis fall within the normal range, it is never a bad idea to try to optimize male fertility potential as much as possible. This process of improving the environment for sperm production starts with the Personal Fertility Profile in Chapter 4. Simple non-invasive measures (such as beginning antioxidant supplementation, quitting smoking, and making healthful changes in lifestyle and diet) are recommended for all couples having difficulty conceiving. More invasive interventions (such as varicocele repair) are typically not recommended in men with normal semen parameters unless other problems were found.
- *Sperm DNA testing.* Chapter 11 reviews advanced sperm testing that can look for elevated levels of DNA fragmenta-

tion (abnormalities in the sperm's genetic material). This type of testing is not routinely recommended for couples who are having trouble conceiving. However, if no problems can be found on standard semen analysis and female fertility testing, it may be useful to check sperm DNA fragmentation levels.

- *Advanced female fertility treatments.* If no problems are found on standard testing of both partners, then a commonly used approach is to begin fertility interventions from the female side, which can potentially increase the odds of conception with each cycle. Options include medications for the female, intrauterine inseminations, and in vitro fertilization. Appendix D discusses the basics of these interventions from the female side.

If a couple proceeds with interventions from the female side, the chances of these interventions being successful are often higher if the man's environment for sperm production is optimized. Often a lot of time, money, and emotion is invested in these interventions, and it makes sense to be sure that the man's semen is as optimal as possible before getting started. I therefore recommend that the male partner proceed with the 10 Week Man Plan in order to increase the couple's overall chances of fertility success.

Unable to Successfully Provide a Specimen for Semen Analysis

For most men, providing a sample for the semen analysis is not something they look forward to doing, but it's not particularly problematic, either. However, some men have trouble producing a semen specimen for testing.

Sometimes men with otherwise normal sexual function are unable to provide a specimen for analysis because of problems with masturbation or an inability to "perform" in the strange environment of a collection room at the fertility lab. This is completely understandable and nothing to be embarrassed about, and it can usually be resolved successfully. Chapter 3 reviews normal collection recommendations as well as suggestions for troubleshooting problems that can occur with specimen collections.

Other men may have a known long-standing problem with erectile dysfunction or ejaculation. Chapter 6 reviews management of erectile dysfunction as well as ejaculation problems.

Recurrent Pregnancy Loss

Sometimes couples do not have an issue with getting pregnant but do have problems with maintaining a pregnancy. The American Society of Reproductive Medicine defines recurrent pregnancy loss as two or more failed pregnancies. After a clinically recognized pregnancy has been established, a woman's chance of losing that pregnancy is about 15–25 percent. Statistically, fewer than five women out of a hundred will have two consecutive pregnancy losses, and only one woman out of a hundred will have three or more consecutive miscarriages.

There are quite a number of factors from the female side that can contribute to pregnancy loss, such as uterine abnormalities, cervical incompetence, blood clotting abnormalities, hormonal issues, infections, immune system problems, and chromosomal abnormalities. Also, the older a woman is, the greater her risk of miscarriage. A thorough evaluation by a fertility specialist is therefore the first step for women suffering from recurrent unexplained pregnancy loss.

A few male-factor issues have also been implicated in elevating the risk of recurrent pregnancy loss. These include chromosomal abnormalities in the father as well as elevated levels of sperm DNA fragmentation. If the results of the woman's evaluation are fairly normal or if miscarriages continue after treatment of the woman, then testing of the male partner is appropriate. This would include checking the man's karyotype (Chapter 10) and sperm DNA testing (Chapter 11).

Recurrent IVF Failure

Even in the best of circumstances, with good-quality embryos, failure rates for a cycle of in vitro fertilization (IVF) approach 50 percent due to persistently low implantation rates. Therefore, every effort should be made to improve sperm quality prior to an IVF cycle to increase the chances of success; start with the Personal Fertility Profile in Chapter 4. Sperm DNA fragmentation testing may be indicated In couples who have failed two or three cycles of IVF for no apparent reason, or those who fail an initial cycle of IVF and had poor embryo quality or progression despite good egg fertilization. There is increasing evidence that elevated levels of sperm DNA fragmentation can contribute to recurrent IVF failure and especially impact embryo quality as well as miscarriage rates. See Chapter 11 for further information regarding testing for sperm DNA abnormalities.

Previous Vasectomy

Approximately half a million vasectomies are performed every year in the United States, and between 3 and 8 percent of these men will change their mind and want to have more children in the future. Effective therapies are available to these men, including microscopic vasectomy reversals as well as sperm extractions combined with conventional in vitro fertilization and intracytoplasmic sperm injection. Chapter 12 reviews these post-vasectomy fertility options in detail.

3

Determining Fertility Potential

This chapter will help men assess their basic fertility potential through semen analysis. It describes how to get an accurate semen analysis performed, and how to interpret the results of this testing.

Getting an Accurate Semen Analysis

The semen analysis represents the foundation of basic male fertility testing. When performed correctly, the semen analysis can provide a wide range of information on male fertility potential as well as point to the presence of important risk factors for infertility.

Because semen varies over time, men with potential fertility problems should not have their assessment of fertility potential based on only one semen analysis. *At least two semen specimens need to be examined, and these specimens need to be checked at least ten weeks apart.* This is because the cycle of spermatogenesis——the production of sperm, from precursor cells to fully mature swimmers— takes around ten weeks, and you want to sample sperm quality from more than one "batch" of sperm that has been produced. So if you have an abnormal semen analysis and your health care provider suggests having another analysis done right away, I would recommend waiting instead, and having the next one done at least ten weeks later. When I see a patient who had two semen analyses done only a few weeks apart, I count the combined results as only one of the needed two analyses.

Choosing the Right Laboratory

When a blood hormone test is performed, the blood is drawn and put into a machine that does automated measurements on the specimen. These measurements are all standardized, so for most fertility-related blood testing it does not matter where you get the tests done. In the vast majority of laboratories, however, semen analyses are performed completely differently. Trained technicians personally evaluate each semen specimen and perform manual measurements, such as counting the sperm (using a specialized counting chamber), deciding how well they are swimming, and assessing whether they have normal shapes. Accuracy depends heavily on how the specimen is handled and processed as well as on the skill of the technician making the measurements.

So where should you have your semen tested?

Most hospital labs provide semen analysis, but the quality of their test results is highly variable. The technicians in hospital laboratories run a huge variety of laboratory tests and do not typically perform semen tests on a daily basis. Comfortable and private collection facilities are often not available, and specimens are not always processed and evaluated in a timely fashion (which can, for example, impact the evaluation of sperm motility). These labs also often do not use the latest diagnostic criteria when assessing the semen. When I see that a semen analysis has been performed at a hospital-based lab, I take the results with a grain of salt. Sperm counts are usually fairly accurate, but other important results, such as motility, morphology, and the presence of elevated levels of white blood cells, are often questionable at best.

By contrast, fertility-specific labs are generally going to provide you with the most accurate evaluation of a semen sample. Fertility-specific labs are typically associated with an IVF group, which offers in vitro fertilization and intrauterine insemination services. This does not mean that you need to make an appointment with an IVF doctor to get testing. Rather, these IVF practices have an associated lab that provides semen testing as a separate service, so when you call to make an appointment for semen analysis, be sure to ask for the lab.

The technicians at fertility-specific labs are highly trained and deal with sperm and fertility-related work exclusively. They generally use the most up-to-date criteria for sperm evaluation. In addition, most fertility-specific labs have private collection rooms with locking doors that are set up to make the experience as comfortable as possible. This eliminates travel time and transport issues with the specimen, which can impact outcomes. Some fertility-specific labs do allow home collections, but under very strict timing and transport guidelines.

There are two ways to locate a nearby fertility-specific laboratory. One is to do an Internet search for local IVF doctors. The second way is to consult the website of the Society for Assisted Reproductive Technology, www.sart.com. This website contains useful information about most IVF clinics in the country. Once on the SART website, click "IVF Success Rates," which will bring you to a map of the country. Use the search engine (by zip code) or click on a state in order to bring up a list of the IVF programs located there. You can then choose a local lab and get its contact information. When you call the clinic, just ask to be transferred to the lab, which can schedule you for a semen analysis.

Cost of a Semen Analysis

Sometimes couples have insurance coverage for semen analysis, but this is highly dependent on individual state regulations as well as the couple's specific insurance policy. Some fertility labs may have contracts with different insurance companies, so testing that is not covered at one facility may be covered at another. Check with your insurance company to verify coverage; give them the test's CPT code (for semen testing, it is V26.21; after October 1, 2015, use Z31.41).

For general reference, the following is a range of prices from several local fertility-specific labs in Ohio for particular tests (with their associated CPT codes):

Semen analysis (not including morphology)	$65–$141	89320
Semen analysis (with morphology)	$125–$268	89320-52
Post-ejaculatory urinalysis	$150–$229	89320-22
Sperm wash (diagnostic)	$135–$268	89261-22
Sperm cryopreservation	$100–$150	89259
Storage of frozen sperm	$180–$360/year	89259
Immunobead testing	$150–$182	89325

If your insurance will cover semen analysis at a local hospital-based lab but not at a fertility-specific lab, I still recommend getting the testing at the fertility-specific lab, as the results will usually be much more accurate and clinically useful. It's worth the extra cost.

Proper Collection Protocol

Once you have identified the lab that you are going to use, you have to follow the proper collection protocol.

Scheduling an Appointment

To allow the laboratory technician adequate time to process and evaluate your specimen, most fertility labs require appointments for semen analysis. Drop-in evaluations are generally not accepted.

The lab will need a semen analysis order that has been signed by your physician, physician assistant, or nurse practitioner. This order can be written on a standard prescription order form; most fertility-specific labs also have their own semen analysis order forms, which can be used as well. A sample semen analysis form can be found in Appendix I of this book, as well as in the "Printable Forms" section of the book's website, www.10weekmanplan.com.

Where the Collection Takes Place

Ideally, the specimen is obtained in a special collection room located at the facility. Fertility-specific labs are typically equipped with such a room to minimize the risk of problems with specimen transport and delivery, although some labs routinely use a home collection protocol. If you do collect at home, make sure that you can get the specimen to the lab *within thirty minutes*. For home collections, it is important to stop by the lab beforehand to pick up the recommended collection cup (I do *not* recommend a do-it-yourself approach to finding a collection container). Once the specimen has been collected at home, it should be sealed in the collection cup, tucked into a pocket to keep it near body temperature, and taken straight to the lab. Home collection specimens need to be prescheduled with the lab, just like specimens collected at the facility.

Abstaining from Sexual Activity Before Collection

The general recommendation is to abstain from sexual activity for two to five days prior to semen analysis. Abstaining for less than two days does not allow the testicles the needed time to build up sperm numbers again after ejaculation. Waiting longer than five days can cause the sperm to "stagnate" and decrease in quality. I generally recommend planning for three or four days of abstinence beforehand, so that if there is a scheduling or timing problem, there is an extra day on either side to keep you in the two-to-five-day window.

Good Aim

Collecting a semen specimen is a new experience for most men and can be quite challenging. Not only do you have to masturbate in an unfamiliar room in an office at a scheduled time, you also have to simultaneously try to collect all of the specimen in a small cup. Most labs supply a collection cup with a wide opening to facilitate the collection process. Problems can still arise, however, and part of the specimen may be lost, which can decrease the accuracy of the results. Practice makes perfect, and it is not a bad idea to "practice" a collection at home into a similar type of cup (like a small paper cup) a week or two prior to your actual semen analysis appointment. I rarely have patients who have problems catching the entire specimen after the first time they try. If you do happen to miss part of the specimen during the "real" collection, be sure to let the lab know, and give them an estimate of approximately what percentage of the ejaculate did not make it into the cup. Also, if you do lose part of the specimen during collection, do not try to scoop up the missed part of the specimen and put it into the cup, or else the analysis may report strange debris and bacteria in your semen.

Lubrication

As if things were not difficult enough already, some labs have you perform your collection by masturbating without any lubrication. Most lubricants (including saliva) are not good for sperm quality and can interfere with accurate evaluation of the specimen. A recent study in the medical journal *Fertility and Sterility* found that the use of isotonic lubricants (those that have roughly the same degree of concentration as other body fluids), such as Pre-Seed, during the collection of a semen analysis specimen did not seem to have any damaging impact on semen parameters. Many labs have begun allowing the use of these isotonic lubricants during specimen collections. If you think you may have a problem collecting without lubrication (which can be tested out at home on your own a few weeks prior), then ask the lab if an isotonic lubricant is okay to use; if it is, ask if they provide this or if you will need to bring your own with you. See "Lubricant Use During Intercourse" in Chapter 6 for a list of lubricants that do not damage sperm quality. Pre-Seed is generally regarded as the best commercially available brand at this time.

Troubleshooting Collection Problems

Unfortunately, some men have significant problems with collecting a specimen for analysis. Some of these men have a long-standing history of erectile dysfunction or ejaculation problems, and for them the difficulties with specimen collection can be anticipated beforehand. For these types of issues, please see the sections "Erectile Dysfunction" and "Ejaculatory Problems" in Chapter 6 for more information.

However, even men with relatively normal sexual function may experience problems with providing a semen specimen for analysis. Potential reasons for this include the inability to collect a specimen in a strange environment, the inability to effectively masturbate in *any* location to collect a specimen, and lack of experience with masturbation.

Inability to Collect a Specimen in a Strange Environment

Most men find the prospect of providing a semen specimen for evaluation a stressful and embarrassing undertaking. Some men just cannot "perform" in a collection room at the lab, whether due to problems with achieving or maintaining an erection or due to difficulty reaching climax.

If the problem is primarily one of achieving or maintaining an erection, sometimes taking an erection-enhancing medication prior to a planned collection may be helpful. For transient sperm collection difficulties in men who normally have fairly good erections, taking 100 mg of Viagra, 20 mg of Levitra or Staxyn, or 20 mg of Cialis one hour prior to the scheduled collection time, or 100 mg of Stendra fifteen to thirty minutes beforehand, may be of benefit. See "Erectile Dysfunction" in Chapter 6 for details on the proper use of these medications, as well as information about side effects and contraindications to taking them.

If collection-related erection problems persist despite use of these medications, or if the primary problem is an inability to reach climax and orgasm in an unfamiliar environment, then collecting a specimen in the comfort of one's home may be helpful. As noted earlier, home collections must be closely coordinated with the lab. Specimens must be kept warm (around body temperature, so keeping them tucked into a pocket is fine) and must make it to the lab within thirty minutes. Also, a proper sterile collection cup must be obtained from the lab prior to specimen collection.

Inability to Effectively Masturbate in Any Location to Collect a Specimen

Some men who have masturbated normally in the past just have a mental block when trying to collect a specimen for evaluation and cannot reach orgasm even in the comfort of their own home. In these situations, sometimes the man's partner needs to get involved to help with collection of the specimen; however, be careful to follow the lab's guidelines regarding allowed lubrication and no use of saliva. Coitus interruptus (having intercourse and then pulling out right before ejaculation) is not recommended: it can be difficult to collect the full specimen, and there is potential for picking up contaminants from the microorganisms normally found in the vagina. A better option is using a special collection condom, which can be then given to the lab technician. Regular condoms *cannot* be used; you must obtain a specially made collection condom beforehand. Ask the lab if it will provide one or if you will need to purchase one on your own. An example of a commercially available collection condom is the Male Factor Pak, which costs around $15. Always check with the lab before using a collection condom to make sure that this is okay with them.

Lack of Experience with Masturbation

Although most men begin masturbating with the onset of puberty, some men make it to adulthood without ever having masturbated. While sociological studies have shown that the vast majority of men (at least 95 percent) masturbate, certain religious groups officially frown upon masturbation, and some men from these religious communities may be unwilling or unable to produce a semen specimen for analysis. Depending on the individual's particular beliefs, a special collection condom (mentioned above) could potentially be used in these circumstances. Working with a local sex therapist can be an effective approach in some situations. Post-coital testing (described at the end of this chapter) can also be used with some couples to see if decent numbers of motile sperm are reaching the cervical mucus, although exact semen parameters cannot be measured.

Planning for IVF with a History of Transient Sperm Collection Problems

If a man has had collection difficulties in the past and his partner is scheduled for an upcoming IVF procedure, I strongly recommend that he collect and freeze sperm well prior to egg retrieval. When eggs are retrieved for IVF, they typically need to be fertilized within about six hours. This can place quite a lot of pressure on a man to "produce" during this six-hour window, especially if the particular IVF lab the couple is using does not offer egg freezing as a last resort. However, if the couple has some backup frozen sperm in reserve, then the pressure is off. In the event that he cannot produce a specimen that day, the frozen sperm can be thawed and used for the IVF cycle, and in most cases the success rate is essentially unchanged.

Semen Analysis Results

The semen analysis is the single most effective measurement tool that we have for predicting male fertility potential, although it's still not perfect. Some men with low sperm counts and poor sperm quality are successful at achieving pregnancies without any medical assistance, while some men with completely normal semen parameters are unable to impregnate a woman. In general, though, in any given population of men, the numbers and quality of sperm present predict rather well whether an otherwise normal couple will have difficulty in establishing a pregnancy.

While semen testing is a powerful tool for evaluating fertility status, it can be hard for patients to interpret the results. This section will discuss normal and abnormal results of semen testing and guide you through understanding your own test results. It will be helpful to have a copy of your latest semen analysis report at hand. I suggest you use the information on it to fill out the chart in Appendix G, My Semen Analysis Parameters. This form can also be found at the book's website, www.10weekmanplan.com, under the "Printable Forms" section.

Information obtained from the standard semen analysis includes:

1. The number of sperm that are present (density)
2. The percentage of sperm that are swimming and how well they are swimming (motility)
3. The percentage of sperm that have normal shapes (morphology)

In addition, the semen analysis can suggest whether blockages, inflammation, or infections may be present.

Variation: When Not to Worry

Many patients are confused and frustrated when they see unexpected differences in their numbers between one semen analysis and another—especially when parameters that seemed normal on an earlier test appear to be going in the wrong direction on a later test. But such differences aren't always something to worry about.

Scientific studies that looked at ejaculations by the same man over a period of time have shown significant week-to-week variation among samples. This natural variability can make accurate determinations of relative fertility or responses to male fertility treatments challenging. In general, I consider about a 20 percent swing in semen parameters to be within the normal expected range of natural variation, a result of the body's sperm production process. Larger swings are more likely to represent a real change in sperm quality for some reason.

	Baseline semen parameters	Normal expected variation on repeat testing	Larger change than would be expected with normal variation
Sperm density	20×10^6/cc	16×10^6/cc to 24×10^6/cc	Less than 16×10^6/cc or more than 24×10^6/cc
Motility	50%	40% to 60%	Less than 40% or more than 60%
Morphology (strict)	5%	4% to 6%	Less than 4% or more than 6%

When questions arise as to whether an observed change is due to natural variation, a real physiologic change, or lab error, additional semen analyses can be helpful in observing general trends over time. For example, if I have a patient who has two semen analyses with markedly different results, I will typically order a third "tie-breaker" analysis at least ten weeks after the second test to get a more accurate picture.

Normal vs. Abnormal

Evaluating semen is not an exact science. To the dismay of people who like to look for concrete answers to problems, there are no specific cut-offs for "fertile" versus "infertile." And while in 2010 the World Health Organization (WHO) published its latest guidelines defining "normal" semen parameters, closer inspection shows that those numbers do not offer clear-cut guidance.

In devising its guidelines, the WHO looked at 4,500 men from fourteen countries and based the "normal" values on a subset of 1,800 men who were able to conceive naturally in less than twelve months. Of these 1,800 men who were able to conceive naturally within a year, the bottom 5 percent of semen parameter values were labeled "abnormal," with the remaining 95 percent of values being labeled "normal."

The following table shows the new 2010 criteria, as well as the previous 1999 criteria for comparison:

	WHO 2010 Criteria	WHO 1999 Criteria
Semen volume	More than 1.5 cc	More than 2.0 cc
Sperm density	15×10^6/cc or more	20×10^6/cc or more
Sperm motility	40% or more	50% or more
Sperm morphology (strict criteria)	4% or more	14% or more
Sperm viability	40% or more	40% or more
White blood cells	Less than 1.0×10^6/cc	Less than 1.0×10^6/cc

As you can see, the latest WHO guidelines define a "normal" sperm density as 15×10^6/cc or more. Let's take a hypothetical man who is trying to have a child. On his semen analysis he is determined to have a sperm count of exactly 15×10^6/cc. Should he feel reassured that his sperm count is within the "normal" range, or should he be troubled that of the men in the WHO study who were able to conceive naturally within a year's time, 95 percent of them had higher sperm counts than he did? Also, 85 percent of men in the WHO study who were *not* able to conceive naturally within a year had sperm counts of at least 15×10^6/cc. Similar comparisons can be made for motility and morphology readings as well. The fact is, *an estimated 50 percent of infertile men have semen parameters that technically fall within the "normal" range* as defined by the WHO criteria.

So how do you sort through all of the controversies associated with defining what is normal and abnormal in terms of semen parameters? In general, the higher a man's overall semen parameters, the better his chances are of successfully establishing a pregnancy by natural intercourse or intra-uterine insemination (IUI). My personal approach is to attempt to optimize sperm count, motility, morphology, and other factors, in order to maximize the couple's chances of conception.

Sperm Density

Sperm density refers to the average number of sperm in a given volume of semen. This is typically referred to as the number (in millions) of sperm per cubic centimeter of ejaculate, and is written as "__ $\times 10^6$/cc." So 20 million sperm per cubic centimeter = 20×10^6/cc. Most people refer to sperm density when discussing sperm counts, although I personally feel that the total motile count (see below) provides a more accurate picture of overall fertility. Normal sperm density in the 2010 WHO guidelines gives a cutoff value of 15×10^6/cc (although I still prefer to use the 1999 edition guidelines of 20×10^6/cc). As discussed later in this chapter, a sperm density of at least 40×10^6/cc may be a more appropriate goal for couples trying to conceive naturally or with insemination.

Terms to Know

A few terms that you might see regarding sperm density include:

- *Oligospermia:* any sperm density that is less than what is considered normal
- *Severe oligospermia:* typically, anything less than 5 million sperm per cubic centimeter (5×10^6/cc)

- *Virtual azoospermia:* when only a very small number of sperm are present in the ejaculate (sometimes defined as less than 100,000 sperm/cc; see Chapter 9)
- *Azoospermia:* no sperm at all seen in the ejaculate (see Chapter 9)

Motility

Sperm motility refers to the percentage of sperm that are swimming. Decreased sperm motility is called asthenospermia.

There are two important parameters to consider when evaluating sperm motility.

- *Total motility:* this denotes the percentage of sperm that are moving. The 2010 WHO guidelines for normal sperm motility are 40 percent or more (although I still prefer to use the 1999 guideline of 50 percent or more).
- Motility grade: this describes how well, on average, the sperm are swimming. This is evaluated on a scale of 0 to 4:

  0   No motility

  1   Sluggish movement with absent or minimal forward progression

  2   Poor to fair activity with forward progression

  3   Good activity with forward progression, tail movement visualized

  4   Full activity, with tail movement difficult to visualize and rapid movement across the field

A normal degree of motility is typically considered to be grade 2 or higher. Sperm with a grade of 0 or 1 are less likely to be able to effectively swim up the fallopian tubes, where egg fertilization occurs.

Different fertility labs use a wide range of methods to report sperm motility. Most labs report only the total percentage of sperm that are swimming and their average motility grade. Some labs report the total percentage of swimming sperm, as well as the percentage of sperm with "progressive" motility. Progressive motility refers to sperm that are moving forward and not just twitching (basically grade 2 or higher). The 2010 WHO guidelines define a normal progressive motility as 32 percent or greater. Some labs will break down what percentage of sperm fall into each motility grade category, for example:

25%	Progressive motility	(Grades 3 and 4)
15%	Slowly progressive	(Grade 2)
10%	Twitching	(Grade 1)
50%	Non-motile	(Grade 0)

One issue to consider regarding motility is the presence of anti-sperm antibodies (ASAs), which can cause sperm to stick together, thereby decreasing their motility (see "Clumping of Sperm and Anti-Sperm Antibodies" in Chapter 6). Most good fertility-specific labs will note on the semen analysis report if significant clumping (also called agglutination) of sperm is seen. Sperm clumping combined with poor motility is suggestive of the presence of ASAs, and their presence can be confirmed on repeat semen analysis with direct (immunobead) ASA testing.

Total Motile Count

Probably the most important predictor of male fertility potential is the total number of swimming sperm that are present in the entire ejaculate. Sperm density only reports the number of sperm present in a milliliter of ejaculate, and ejaculate volumes can vary widely. A man with a sperm density of 30×10^6/cc with an ejaculate volume of 1.1 cc has the same number of total swimming sperm as a man with a sperm density of 6.6×10^6/cc and an ejaculate volume of 5.0 cc (assuming equivalent sperm motility for both), even though the sperm density was normal for the first man and significantly abnormal for the second man.

The total motile count (TMC) gets around this problem by combining the sperm density, motility, and ejaculate volumes to provide the total number of swimming sperm that are present in the entire ejaculate. Given the importance of the TMC, it is surprising that many fertility labs do not report it as part of the semen analysis.

Some labs do report TMC but call it "total motile sperm," "motile sperm count," or some other similar variation. The key to identifying what the lab is talking about is the unit of measure. For TMC it should say "million" (or "__× 10^6"), as opposed to "millions per cc" (or "__ × 10^6/cc") for sperm density. Another measure you may see is "total count," which is the total number of both swimming and non-motile sperm; this is not as clinically useful as TMC.

If the TMC is not reported, it can be easily calculated by using the following equation:

(Ejaculated Volume × Sperm Density × Total Motility) ÷ 100 = TMC

For example, if ejaculate volume is 2.0 cc, sperm density is 30×10^6/cc, and total motility is 50 percent, the TMC is (2.0 × 30 × 50) ÷ 100 = 30 million sperm.

In terms of successfully establishing a pregnancy with natural intercourse or intrauterine insemination, higher numbers of total swimming sperm are better. A TMC of 20 million sperm is getting into the territory of good fertility potential, while a completely normal TMC is typically considered to be 75 million sperm or higher (see box). A minimum TMC of 5 million sperm is typically considered the lower cutoff for IUI.

Where Does the "Normal" TMC Come From?

How did a TMC of 75 million sperm or higher come to be considered "normal"? That figure is based on two studies that looked at natural pregnancy rates and sperm density.

The first looked at 430 couples and their chances of establishing a pregnancy within six months of starting natural intercourse. The study, conducted by J. P. Bonde and colleagues and published in the *Lancet* in October 1998, found that chances of pregnancy increased as the man's sperm density approached 40×10^6/cc, but that above 40×10^6/cc the odds did not improve further.

The second study, carried out by R. Slama and colleagues and published in *Human Reproduction* in February 2002, looked at 940 couples who achieved pregnancy naturally and found a correlation between decreasing time to achieve pregnancy and rising sperm counts up to 55×10^6/cc; after that level, pregnancy did not occur more quickly.

The conclusion we can reach from these studies is that sperm densities of 40 to 55×10^6/cc may improve the chances of natural pregnancy. I tend to be a little conservative and use as a goal the lower sperm density cited in the first study mentioned above (40×10^6/cc). In this study, the average semen volume was 3.14 cc and the average motility was 61.4 percent. Plugging these figures into the equation for calculating TMC produces $(3.14 \times 40 \times 61.4) \div 100 = 77 \times 10^6$ sperm. The studies showed an increasing chance of natural conception up to this level, but no significant further improvement with higher TMC numbers.

You should be aware that this interpretation of a "normal" TMC may be controversial, and other male fertility experts may have other definitions of a normal range. However, I feel that the available studies suggest that a goal of at least 75 million swimming sperm is reasonable.

One very important consideration to keep in mind when evaluating TMC is the average motility grade. If most of the sperm are only twitching, then their fertility potential is not going to be very good for natural intercourse or IUI. Therefore, a TMC is considered normal only if the average grade of motility is 2 or higher.

How do you calculate TMC if the lab has broken down the percentage of sperm with each different motility grade? Do you include the grade 1 (twitching) sperm in the calculation of total moving sperm? There is no absolutely correct answer to this. I tend to include the total motility (all grades 1 through 4) in the TMC calculation, as this was how it was done in the studies that established the "normal" sperm density cutoffs of 40–55 × 10⁶ sperm.

Morphology

No other part of the semen analysis generates such controversy and difference of opinion as does the sperm morphology reading. Morphology refers to the percentage of sperm with perfectly normal shapes. Morphology readings assess multiple aspects of a sperm's shape, including its head, midpiece, and tail, as well as the presence of cytoplasmic droplets. Abnormal sperm morphology is called teratospermia. Because of the highly subjective nature of morphology readings, I typically only take into consideration morphology findings from fertility-specific laboratories, not hospital-based labs.

Traditionally, there have been two main sets of guidelines that are thought to be potentially clinically useful in terms of morphology: the WHO guidelines (third edition) and the Kruger strict morphology guidelines. (To make things more complicated, the WHO has issued a fourth edition of its guidelines that essentially follow the Kruger strict morphology guidelines. For simplicity, when I refer to the WHO guidelines, I will be referring to the third edition guidelines.)

The WHO guidelines require 30 percent or more normal forms for a result of "normal." Note that it is quite common to see WHO morphology readings of 5 percent or lower, but very rare to see a WHO reading of 40 percent or greater (at least in tests by accurate fertility-specific labs).

What are known as the Kruger strict criteria were developed in 1986 by a physician named Thinus Kruger and were based upon the evaluation of sperm that had successfully migrated to the cervix following natural intercourse. The original 1986 guidelines used a figure of 14 percent or greater normal forms as the cutoff for "normal" morphology. However, the strictness of the guidelines has changed over the years, and many labs now use 4 percent or more as the new definition of "normal" (as do the latest WHO guidelines). I too use the 4 percent figure as the lower limit of "normal," although many of the labs in my area still print the higher 14 percent guideline on their official semen analysis reports (a source of endless confusion and anxiety for my patients).

There are some other morphology criteria that you may occasionally see used by hospital labs, such as those of the American Society of Clinical Pathology (ASCP). I have not found these to be clinically useful and do not give them any consideration. Instead, I recommend repeat testing at a fertility-specific lab that can provide an accurate strict morphology evaluation.

Importance of Morphology

Various studies over the years have looked at the relationship between sperm morphology and pregnancy outcomes with natural intercourse, intrauterine insemination (IUI), and in-vitro fertilization (IVF). However, these studies are often contradictory and do not provide a clear picture of the impact of sperm morphology.

One important consideration to keep in mind when looking at morphology is simple statistics. A semen specimen can have over 100 million sperm in the sample, but only two hundred of these sperm—or 0.0002 percent—are typically evaluated in order to calculate a Kruger strict morphology. When I see two reports showing 4 percent normal forms in one and 2 percent in the other, it is difficult for me to be confident that there is a significant clinical difference, as I know how small the sample size is.

In terms of natural intercourse and IUI, I find the Kruger strict morphology by itself is a fairly weak predictor of how easily a pregnancy can be established. That being said, I think that it is worthwhile for couples who are having problems conceiving to take steps to try to improve the Kruger strict morphology results as much as possible. But even if the Kruger strict morphology value is 0 percent, the chance of pregnancy is still usually decent as long as the sperm counts and motility are normal. For couples considering IUI, if the TMC is good, then I do not think that a low morphology should necessarily preclude a trial of IUI rather than just jumping straight to IVF; however, if the Kruger strict morphology value is very low, perhaps they should try just two or three cycles of IUI, rather than four, before moving on to IVF. For couples considering IVF, I tell them that there are good data suggesting that if the strict morphology is very low (less than 4 percent), then intracytoplasmic sperm injection (ICSI) should be used instead of standard IVF.

Abnormal Morphology and Birth Defects

A common question I hear from couples is that if a morphologically abnormal sperm fertilizes an egg, will the resulting child have a higher chance of having a birth defect or health problem? I feel comfortable reassuring them that the answer to this is generally no, there is no increased risk.

Levels of sperm DNA fragmentation do not seem to correlate well with strict morphology readings (see Chapter 11 for more information on sperm DNA testing). Some studies have shown that the DNA of morphologically abnormal sperm do tend to have increased rates of certain types of genetic flaws (called aneuploidy). However, this does not seem to translate into a higher risk of genetic or physical abnormalities in the offspring. There are likely two reasons for this. First, the unfertilized egg contains very efficient screening mechanisms for weeding out defective sperm and preferentially letting normal sperm through its outer layers to start the fertilization process. Second, nature seems to be very efficient at identifying embryos with genetic abnormalities and not allowing them to progress. These mechanisms are not 100 percent efficient, but rates of health problems and birth defects do not seem to be higher in the children of men with lower morphology readings, whether the pregnancy was established by natural intercourse, IUI, or standard IVF.

Some concern does exist as to whether there is an increased risk of birth defects when ICSI is used with IVF (see Appendix D), since with this technique the eggs' natural screening mechanisms are bypassed, potentially allowing through a higher percentage of sperm with defective DNA. However, nature's efficiency at removing genetically defective embryos has led to the vast majority of ICSI babies being born completely healthy and normal.

Globozoospermia

There is a rare type of teratospermia called globozoospermia in which all of the sperm in the sample have small round heads and lack an acrosome cap. The acrosome cap is an enzyme-filled structure covering the front part of the head of the sperm; it helps penetrate the outer layer of the egg to allow the sperm's DNA to enter. Sperm that lack an acrosome cap are unable to fertilize an egg without the use of ICSI, an IVF technique in which a sperm is directly injected into an egg. Another problem is that even when ICSI is utilized, fertilization rates using sperm from men with globozoospermia tend to be very low, for reasons that have not been fully explained. Specialized IVF laboratory techniques, such as assisted oocyte activation (AOA), have been found to improve fertilization rates in some of these cases.

True globozoospermia is a genetic problem and cannot be reversed. I sometimes see patients whose first semen analysis indicates that the sperm sampled have absolutely no acrosome caps, but on repeat analysis, after the environment for sperm production has been optimized, sperm with acrosome caps are present. However, if multiple semen analyses show complete globozoospermia, then ICSI with a technique such as AOA likely offers the best chance to establish a pregnancy. Another option in this situation would be to use donor sperm (see Appendix F).

Ejaculate Volume

The role of the semen is to efficiently transport sperm to the cervix while protecting them from the harsh, acidic environment of the vagina. A standard semen analysis almost always includes an assessment of ejaculate volume, color, and time for liquefaction. Some labs will also routinely check pH and sometimes semen fructose. These semen parameters will make more sense if you know the relative contributions of the testicles, seminal vesicles, and prostate to the ejaculate fluid.

- *Testicles: 0.1 cc.* The testicles supply the sperm and a small amount of fluid (about 5–10 percent of the total ejaculate volume). Because this is such a small percentage of total volume, men who have had a vasectomy, in which the flow of fluid from the testicles is blocked, do not notice any difference in ejaculate volume.

- *Seminal vesicles: 1.5 cc, alkaline pH.* The seminal vesicles supply the bulk of the fluid volume (about 65–70 percent). Seminal vesicle fluid causes the ejaculate to coagulate, and also provides fructose as an energy source for the sperm. Since the majority of fluid comes from the seminal vesicles, the overall pH of a normal ejaculate is alkaline.

- *Prostate: 0.5 cc, acidic pH.* The prostate gland produces around 25–30 percent of seminal fluid. Prostatic fluid provides enzymes that cause the coagulated semen to liquefy, thereby releasing the sperm into the cervical mucus. Typically, the ejaculate liquefies completely within twenty to thirty minutes when evaluated in the lab.

- *Bulbourethral glands (Cowper's glands).* The bulbourethral glands are pea-sized glands, located at the base of the penis, that open into the urethra. With arousal, these glands produce a small amount of a clear, salty, viscous secretion called pre-ejaculate. The pre-ejaculate serves to lubricate the urethra and neutralize any acidic urine that may remain within the urethra from the last urination. Although the bulbourethral glands do not typically serve as a reservoir for sperm, their fluid can pick up sperm dwelling within the urethra from the last ejaculation and carry them out.

The latest WHO criteria list a normal ejaculate volume as greater than 1.5 cc. However, I personally use 1.0 cc as the cutoff for what I consider normal, since in my clinical experience I have found extremely low rates of ejaculatory problems (such as retrograde ejaculation) in men with ejaculate volumes between 1.1 cc and 1.5 cc. See Chapter 6 for more information on the interpretation of semen volume results.

Semen pH and Fructose

In normal circumstances, the pH of the ejaculate is alkaline (a pH greater than 7.5), since the alkaline fluid from the seminal vesicles makes up the largest part of the ejaculate. The seminal vesicles also produce fructose. So when the ejaculate has an alkaline pH and contains fructose, it indicates that fluid from the seminal vesicles is making it into the ejaculate.

Semen Color

This assessment is highly subjective and rarely clinically useful. One exception is with complete ejaculatory obstruction, where the semen is often entirely clear.

Semen Liquefaction and Viscosity

The fluid from the seminal vesicles causes sperm to coagulate, in order to hold the sperm near the cervical opening and protect them from the harsh vaginal environment. The enzymes in the prostatic fluid then cause the sperm to gradually liquefy, facilitating release of the sperm into the cervical canal. The rate at which the semen liquefies is often measured as viscosity (normal is less than 2) or liquefaction time (normal liquefaction times range from five to twenty-five minutes, with an average around twenty minutes; times of more than thirty minutes are considered abnormal).

White Blood Cells or Round Cells

All men have some white blood cells (WBCs) present within their semen, as these cells play a role in maintaining a good, healthy environment for sperm. However, elevated levels of WBCs can be a marker of inflammation or infection. When too many WBCs are seen in the sperm, it is called pyospermia. Normal levels of WBCs are generally considered to be either 1 million/cc or less *or* 10–15/hpf or less (some labs refer to the number of WBCs seen per high power field, or hpf, when observed under a tabletop microscope).

The diagnosis of pyospermia is complicated by the fact that under a microscope, WBCs resemble immature sperm cells. Thus, there can be confusion when these cells are counted, leading to incorrect WBC counts. Immature sperm cells do not directly impact fertility, but they are often found in higher numbers in men with sperm production problems and low sperm counts.

Many labs report the number of "round cells," which can include both WBCs and immature sperm cells. Statistically speaking, when male fertility patients have elevated numbers of round cells, two-thirds of the time it is because of higher levels of immature sperm cells, and about one-third of the time it is because of abnormally high levels of white blood cells.

Standard staining methods used by most non-fertility-specific labs (for example, Giemsa and Papanicolaou stains) cannot reliably differentiate WBCs from immature sperm cells. Most fertility-specific labs use specialized techniques to differentiate the two types of round cells. Immunohistochemical techniques are the gold standard; this is a labor-intensive and costly process that uses monoclonal antibodies to detect all three types of white blood cells (granulocytes, macrophages, and T lymphocytes). A peroxidase stain is a quick and inexpensive technique that only detects granulocytes, but since these represent the most common type of white blood cell found in the semen, it is felt to be sufficient for clinical purposes. A Wright stain is a histologic stain that is often used in the differentiation of blood cell types.

It is important to be able to differentiate between elevated levels of immature sperm cells (which are not clinically significant) and pyospermia (which can often have a detrimental impact on sperm function). My recommendation is that if a lab reports only an elevated number of round cells, you should obtain a follow-up analysis at a fertility-specific lab that offers one of the techniques needed to see if pyospermia is truly present.

Other Sperm Testing

Post-Coital Testing

The post-coital test (PCT) involves evaluating the cervical mucus microscopically following intercourse for the presence of sperm. A

PCT must be performed in the peri-ovulatory period (when the cervical mucus is most receptive to sperm), and the testing is done approximately two to eight hours after intercourse.

PCT is not commonly performed, but can be potentially useful when there is concern regarding sperm delivery to the cervical mucus. Reasons for ordering PCT testing include:

- Hyperviscous (extra-thick) semen
- Unexplained infertility
- Low volume of ejaculate with normal sperm count
- Evaluating the fertility potential of men who are not able to produce a specimen by masturbation or with a special collection condom
- Concerns about cervical problems
- Proximal hypospadias (an abnormality in the position of the urethral opening of the penis) when there are concerns that sperm are not being deposited near the cervix

A normal test result is when more than 10 sperm are seen per high power field (hpf) under the microscope.

Rarely Used Sperm Tests

Other fertility tests that are not used much anymore include tests that can evaluate the interaction between sperm and egg: capacitation (biochemical changes within the sperm when it enters the female reproductive tract that allow it to fertilize an egg); acrosome reaction (a release of enzymes from the acrosome cap that allows the sperm to penetrate the egg and initiate fertilization); and sperm zona binding (which tests the ability of the sperm to attach to the zona pellucida).

In the pre-ICSI era, these tests provided potentially important information, as only standard IVF was available, in which sperm were mixed with an egg in a sterile laboratory dish and the sperm and egg had to interact normally. However, the ability to perform ICSI, in which a single sperm is injected directly into an egg, has made the determination of egg-sperm interactions less important.

It is unlikely that you will encounter any of these tests during your fertility evaluation. However, your health care provider may order them in select circumstances.

4

Developing a Personal Fertility Profile

Most couples are interested in developing an efficient and effective plan that optimizes their chances of conception by focusing on only those factors that are relevant to them. The 10 Week Man Plan utilizes a Personal Fertility Profile to help couples develop an individualized strategy for managing male factor fertility issues. Completing it will help guide you toward the information that will be most valuable for your particular situation.

Completing the Profile

The Personal Fertility Plan helps to identify the specific male factors that may be preventing a couple from achieving their fertility goals.

First, fill out the My Semen Analysis Parameters form (in Appendix G of this book, or downloadable from the "Printable Forms" section of the book's website, www.10weekmanplan.com). If you've read Chapter 3, you may have already filled it out; if not, fill it out now. You'll need to have copies of your latest two or three semen analysis reports in order to complete that form.

Next you'll fill out the Personal Fertility Profile (in Appendix H of this book, or downloadable from the "Printable Forms" section of www.10weekmanplan.com). The information needed in Section 1 of this form will come from the My Semen Analysis Parameters form. Then fill out Sections 2 through 7 (Demographics, Lifestyle, Job-Related Issues, Medications and Supplements, Past Medical History, and Sexual History).

The next step is to have a fertility-specific physical examination performed by a physician, physician assistant, or nurse practitioner (see the next section, "Fertility-Related Physical Exam"). This information can then be used to fill in Section 8 of the Personal Fertility Profile.

The last step is to have hormone testing done. This will need to be ordered by your health care provider. The section "Hormone Testing in Men" later in this chapter reviews the importance of hormones to male fertility and discusses how to determine which hormone tests are appropriate for you. The results of the hormone testing can then be used to fill in Section 9 of the Personal Fertility Profile.

Fertility-Related Physical Exam

A physical exam performed by your health care provider is an important part of the fertility evaluation. Obviously, the parts of the exam relating to the penis and testicles are the most pertinent to fertility, and these areas will be the focus of this section.

Usually all that's needed is a manual and visual check by a physician, physician assistant, or nurse practitioner. Sometimes, though, it is difficult to check the scrotum adequately. This can be because of extreme patient sensitivity and/or pain on examination of this area. Significant obesity may also make it difficult to do an adequate physical examination. And on occasion a large hydrocele (collection of fluid around the testicle) may prohibit the physician from adequately palpating the epididymis and testicle. In these circumstances, a scrotal ultrasound can be ordered for a better look.

Specifics of the Male Physical Exam

Some couples may prefer to leave the details of the exam to their health care provider. However, for those couples interested in a more in-depth discussion of the various aspects of the physical exam, this section can serve as a guide to what the doctor is looking for on the evaluation.

Testicles

Two Testicles, One on Each Side

It is important to make sure that a testicle can be felt on each side. If a testicle is not palpable, then a reason for this should be found. Reasons may include a history of an undescended testicle that was not repaired, retractile testicles, neonatal testicular torsion, or surgical removal of a testicle.

Size and Consistency of the Testicle

Ninety-five percent of the volume of the testicles is made up by the cells that produce sperm. Therefore, a normal-size testicle is often a sign that sperm production is not severely impaired. (However, this is not always the case; see, for example, "Maturation Arrest" in Chapter 9.) Small, firm testicles often indicate a problem with sperm production that occurred before the onset of puberty (such as Klinefelter's disease). Small, soft testicles are typically more consistent with sperm production problems that developed after puberty.

Testicular volume can be measured in one of several ways. One is to measure the testicles' dimensions—length, width, and height—and plug those into a formula:

$$\text{Volume} = 4/3\pi \times (\text{length}/2) \times (\text{width}/2) \times (\text{height}/2)$$

Calipers can also be used to approximate the dimensions, although estimates can vary somewhat depending on how tightly the physician stretches the scrotal skin over the testicle as the measurements are taken.

Normal testicular dimensions are:

Length: 3–5 cm

Width: 2–4 cm

Height: 3 cm

Normal testicular volume is about 20 cm^3, with a range of 15 to 25 cm^3. (The units you see on a report may vary, but cubic centimeters, which are abbreviated as *cm^3* or *cc*, are the same as milliliters, which are abbreviated *mL*: 1 cm^3 = 1 cc = 1 mL.)

It is far easier to estimate the testicular volume using an orchidometer, which is a series of plastic beads of different sizes looped together on a string. Each bead is labeled with its volume in cubic centimeters or milliliters. The beads are held up alongside the scrotum during the physical exam to get an estimation of the testicular volume. As with the use of calipers, there is some subjectivity involved in measurement with an orchidometer, depending on how tightly the physician stretches the scrotal skin over the testicle while making the measurement. Normal testicular volumes generally range from 12 cc to 20 cc.

The most accurate way to measure testicular volume is with ultrasound. However, ultrasound testing can cost several hundred dollars, and most fertility patients do not need their testicular volume determined this accurately. In some circumstances, such as adolescents who have varicoceles, testicular volumes are followed over time to see if treatment is needed for the testicles to develop properly, and using ultrasound to track testicular volumes precisely over time makes sense with these patients. However, in the majority of adult male fertility patients, an approximate estimation of testicular volume is all that's needed.

Testicular Masses

Testicular cancer occurs in higher rates in men with fertility problems. An abnormal testicular mass found on examination should be evaluated further with ultrasound.

Scrotal Skin Abnormalities

Genital warts (caused by the human papillomavirus, or HPV) are a fairly common form of sexually transmitted disease. Certain types of HPV have been associated with an increased risk of penile cancer in men and cervical cancer in women. If genital warts are found, they should be treated by ablative therapy (such as topical creams, laser ablation, etc.). These treatments do not permanently cure the man of HPV, but they can remove visible lesions and decrease (although not eliminate) the risk of spread to sexual partners. Female partners should have regular Pap smears with their gynecologist to look for abnormal cervical changes that might need further evaluation and treatment.

Epididymis

Present in Full on Both Sides

The epididymis, the structure on the side of the testicles in which the sperm mature, has three parts: the head, body, and tail. In congenital bilateral absence of the vas deferens, the body and tail of the epididymis can be missing, resulting in obstruction.

No Masses

Cysts of the epididymis are quite common. In men of reproductive age, these cysts are usually relatively small and asymptomatic. On rare occasions, epididymal cysts can be associated with chronic discomfort in the scrotum. Occasionally they can also grow to be very large (grapefruit size or larger) and make sitting uncomfortable. By themselves, epididymal cysts generally do not cause fertility problems unless they are very large. However, surgical removal of these cysts can cause epididymal scarring, which can lead to obstruction problems.

Tumors of the epididymis are rare, and the majority that are found are benign, not cancerous. Therefore, when an asymptomatic mass that is clearly coming from the epididymis (not the testicle) is discovered, it is usually a cyst, and generally these do not need to be imaged by ultrasound. All men of reproductive age should do regular scrotal exams every few months in the shower. If any significant changes are noted with an epididymal mass over time, such as an increase in size, then ultrasound imaging is recommended. Also, if there is significant pain associated with an epididymal mass, then an ultrasound should also be performed.

Fullness or Congestion

A skilled health care professional should be able to determine if the epididymis feels swollen or congested. This can be consistent with a blockage of sperm transport, with sperm backing up into the epididymis and causing congestion. Congenital epididymal obstruction and previous vasectomy are two potential causes of this finding (see Chapter 9). Epididymal swelling can also be due to inflammation or infection within the epididymis.

Tenderness

The nerve supply for the testicle enters around the area of the head of the epididymis. Due to its rich nerve supply, the epididymis is often somewhat tender to the touch during a physical exam. However, extra tenderness can also be due to inflammation within the epididymis itself (epididymitis).

Spermatic Cord

The spermatic cord contains the blood supply, nerves, and lymphatic drainage for the testicles. It also contains the vas deferens, which is a tube-like structure that carries the sperm to the ejaculatory ducts. In patients with congenital bilateral absence of the vas deferens (CBAVD), the vas deferens is typically missing on both sides. A vas deferens that is not palpable on only one side can either represent an atypical variant of CBAVD or be part of a mesonephric duct abnormality, affecting also the kidney and ureter on that side (see Chapter 10 for more information on CBAVD).

Varicoceles

Dilated veins in the scrotum are called varicoceles; they are similar to varicose veins in the legs. Small varicoceles are not clinically significant, but larger varicoceles can have a negative impact on sperm production and quality. Most varicoceles can be diagnosed by examining the man while he is standing. When a man with a varicocele increases his intra-abdominal pressure (by performing what is called a Valsalva maneuver—it's usually done by closing your mouth and pinching your nose shut, then trying to exhale), the doctor can usually feel what's called an impulse within the dilated veins.

Varicoceles are classified on the following scale:

Subclinical: the varicocele can be seen on ultrasound but not felt on physical exam.

Grade 1: An impulse can be felt on Valsalva maneuver, but the veins do not feel dilated in size on exam.

Grade 2: Scrotal veins feel dilated on examination, and an impulse is felt on Valsalva maneuver.

Grade 3: Scrotal veins are enlarged to the point where they can be seen through the scrotal skin with just a visual inspection. These dilated veins typically are described as feeling like a "bag of worms" on physical examination.

Subclinical and Grade 1 varicoceles are typically not considered clinically significant, whereas Grades 2 and 3 varicoceles are potentially a cause of decreased semen parameters.

Sometimes a physical exam reveals a varicocele that is borderline in size. In other circumstances, a good evaluation of the veins cannot be obtained, either because of extreme obesity or because the patient experiences sensitivity or discomfort with deep palpation in the scrotal area. In these situations, a scrotal ultrasound can be performed, measuring the diameter of the largest scrotal veins while the man is in a standing position. Veins that are larger than 3.5 mm in size are considered potentially clinically significant. See the "Varicoceles" section in Chapter 6 for more information.

Penis

Normal Size and Location of Meatus

The meatus (opening) of the penis is typically located at the tip of the penile head. However, in men with hypospadias or epispadias, the location of the meatus can be elsewhere on the penis, or even in the perineal region (the area of skin between the penis and scrotum). If the meatus is located near the head of the penis, then there is unlikely to be any significant impact on fertility. However, if the meatus is not near the head of the penis, then during intercourse the sperm are likely not being deposited near the woman's cervix, which can have a significant impact on the ability to establish a pregnancy naturally. This problem can often be overcome by collecting the sperm during ejaculation and using it in conjunction with intrauterine insemination (see Appendix D).

Presence or Absence of Discharge

A discharge of fluid from the opening of the penis can be a sign of infection within the urethra or genital duct system.

Presence or Absence of Skin Abnormalities

As with the scrotum, genital warts, caused by HPV, are relatively common. See the "Scrotal Skin Abnormalities" section above for more information on genital warts.

Hormone Testing in Men

Hormones play a vital role in maintaining normal sperm production as well as male sexual function and hormone imbalances are a relatively common cause of fertility and sexual problems in men.

Who Should Get Hormone Testing?

Any man whose fertility testing has revealed any abnormality should have his hormones tested. This includes men with abnormal semen parameters (volume, density, motility, morphology) as well as men with abnormal results on sperm DNA testing.

In addition, men with symptoms of low testosterone should get hormonal testing for hypogonadism (also called "low T"), a condition in which the body doesn't produce enough testosterone. These symptoms can include:

- Erectile dysfunction
- Decreased libido (sex drive)
- Decreased energy or motivation
- Low mood or decreased feelings of well-being
- Decreased intensity of orgasm
- Difficulty achieving orgasm
- Decreased ejaculate volume
- Increased fat deposits around the abdomen

- Decreased muscle mass
- Osteoporosis or osteopenia (increased bone fragility)

What Initial Hormone Testing Should Be Ordered?

A general hormone panel for all men with fertility issues should include:

- Total testosterone and bioavailable (or free) testosterone. (Because free testosterone levels can vary depending on the technique the lab uses to measure them, it may be better to check levels of bioavailable testosterone, unless you are working with an infertility specialist who is comfortable with interpreting the results. See "Interpretation of Hormone Testing Results," below, for more details.)
- Luteinizing hormone (LH)
- Estradiol

Your health care provider may order other tests as necessary:

- Follicle-stimulating hormone (FSH); recommended for men with low sperm density or low total motile sperm count
- Thyroid-stimulating hormone (TSH); recommended if there are symptoms that may indicate an underactive thyroid (including fatigue, cold intolerance, sleepiness, weight gain, muscle aches, abnormally slow heart rate, constipation, dry skin, brittle hair, decreased concentration or memory) or an overactive thyroid (including nervousness, fatigue, weakness, palpitations, heat intolerance, excessive sweating, diarrhea, insomnia, poor concentration, weight loss, abnormally fast heart rate, and warm and moist skin)

Role of Hormones in Male Fertility

Gonadotropins

The part of the brain called the hypothalamus plays a critical role in a man's hormonal system. The hypothalamus produces gonadotropin-releasing hormone (GnRH), which stimulates the nearby pituitary gland. The pituitary gland regulates multiple organ systems, but from a male fertility standpoint, the pituitary produces two important gonadotropins, or hormones that act on the reproductive system: LH and FSH.

LH travels via the bloodstream to the testicles, where it stimulates the Leydig cells to produce testosterone. FSH also travels through the bloodstream to the testicles, where it stimulates the spermatogenic cells as well as the Sertoli (support) cells, both of which play a part in sperm production.

Testosterone

Testosterone is an androgen—a substance that binds to particular receptors in the body's cells and produces masculine characteristics. There are several kinds of natural androgens, but the body breaks them all down into testosterone. Under normal circumstances, most androgens in a man's body are produced by the Leydig cells within the testicles in response to LH secreted by the pituitary gland. (A small part of the total amount of androgens—less than 10 percent—is produced by the adrenal glands, which sit above the kidneys.)

When the testicles are functioning normally, high levels of intra-testicular testosterone are maintained which is necessary for optimal sperm production. The testosterone then finds its way into the bloodstream, where it is required for other normal bodily functions, including getting and maintaining an erection, sex drive, and bone health. The amount of testosterone in the bloodstream is detected by the pituitary, and normally when the testosterone drops below a certain level, the pituitary secretes more LH, which in turn tells the testicles to produce more testosterone.

This feedback loop works correctly only when the testosterone circulating in the bloodstream has been produced by the testicles themselves (what's called endogenous testosterone production). When testosterone is given to a man directly—for example, as testosterone replacement therapy or as anabolic steroids—these exogenous androgens raise the blood levels of testosterone, tricking the brain into thinking that the testicles do not need to make any more testosterone. LH secretion from the pituitary decreases, and testosterone production by the testicles decreases dramatically. Blood testosterone levels (which we can directly measure with blood testing) remain high, but testicular testosterone levels (which we cannot measure clinically without direct aspiration) become very low, and this can result in significant decreases in sperm production.

Estradiol

Estradiol is a sex hormone with estrogenic (feminizing) actions that is found in both men and women. In women, estradiol is made by the ovaries and plays an important role in the female reproductive process. In men, the role of this hormone in maintaining general health has not been completely defined, but estradiol is known to play a significant part (along with testosterone) in maintaining normal bone strength. Since men do not have ovaries, they obtain about 80 percent of their estradiol through an enzyme called aromatase (found primarily in the testicles, liver, and fat cells), which converts a certain percentage of a man's testosterone into estradiol; the remaining 20 percent of a man's estradiol appears to be produced directly by the testicles.

In men, if estradiol levels get too high or become out of balance with the testosterone, it can have a negative impact on sperm production. Elevated estradiol levels can also lead to abnormal enlargement of male breast tissue, called gynecomastia. A common misconception is that elevated estradiol levels can counteract the sexual effects of testosterone, leading to such symptoms as decreased libido and erectile dysfunction. However, recent studies have shown that normal estradiol levels may in fact play an important role in maintaining normal male sexual function, while very low estradiol levels can actually contribute to problems of low libido in some men. Decreased estradiol levels have also been correlated with increases in body fat and decreased bone health. In contrast, lower testosterone levels tend to lead to symptoms such as decreased lean body mass, decreased muscle size and strength, and increased bone weakness. Further studies will need to be performed to pinpoint the relative contributions of estradiol and testosterone in men.

Prolactin

Prolactin, a peptide hormone made by the pituitary gland, has multiple functions throughout the body; it may be best known for its role in stimulating lactation in women. In men, mild increases in prolactin do not seem to cause infertility and should not be treated. However, significantly elevated levels of prolactin (hyperprolactinemia) can inhibit GnRH release from the hypothalamus, which in turn can result in a decrease in FSH and LH release. In men, this drop in gonadotropin release can decrease testosterone levels and cause problems with sperm production and quality.

Thyroid-Stimulating Hormone (TSH)

The thyroid gland sits in the lower part of the neck and produces hormones that are involved in the regulation of the body's metabolic rate. The two thyroid hormones, thyroxine (T4) and triiodothyronine (T3), serve to increase the body's metabolic rate by stimulating enzymatic reactions involved in the metabolism of carbohydrates, fats, and proteins. Abnormalities in thyroid hormone production include overproduction (hyperthyroidism) and underproduction (hypothyroidism). Both are diagnosed by an elevation or decrease in TSH (thyroid-stimulating hormone), which is produced by the pituitary gland. Thyroid problems are a relatively rare cause of male infertility, but when severe, both hyperthyroidism and hypothyroidism can result in problems with sperm production and sperm quality in some men.

Inhibin B

Inhibin B is a glycoprotein hormone produced predominately by the Sertoli cells within the testicles; it is involved in the feedback process that regulates the formation of sperm. When it reaches the pituitary gland via the bloodstream, inhibin causes a decrease in FSH secretion. When sperm production is normal, inhibin maintains normal (i.e., low) FSH levels. However, when sperm production is compromised, the Sertoli cells decrease their production of inhibin, which results in increased FSH production by the pituitary gland, to drive the testicles to make more sperm.

In some ways, inhibin may represent a better indicator of sperm production than FSH, since it is a direct marker produced by the testicles (as opposed to FSH, which is an indirect marker produced by the pituitary gland). However, inhibin has not been studied nearly as extensively as FSH, testing for it is more expensive, and the test has some of the same diagnostic limitations as FSH (such as false normal values in some azoospermic men with maturation arrest; see Chapter 9 for more details).

Androgen replacement therapy can cause inhibin levels can decrease, but typically not to undetectable levels. HCG injections do not seem to have an impact on inhibin levels. FSH injections at modest levels also do not seem to directly impact inhibin levels, but higher dosages of FSH may cause them to rise. Clomiphene (used to treat certain hormonal abnormalities in men; see Chapter 7) does not appear to have a significant impact on inhibin levels under normal circumstances, but this has not been extensively studied; in contrast, clomiphene does cause elevations in FSH levels because of its impact on estrogen receptors on the pituitary gland.

Recommendations for Hormone Testing

I always recommend that my patients get baseline hormone levels tested before starting hormonal medications (such as clomiphene, anastrozole, or HCG; see Chapter 7). Unfortunately, it is quite common for some physicians to prescribe these medications based on a semen analysis without first checking baseline hormone levels to see if there's even a need for them. Medications such as clomiphene seem to be effective only if there is a hormone abnormality that needs to be corrected; they generally won't improve semen parameters by themselves if hormone levels are normal.

Timing of Hormone Testing

Blood for most types of hormone testing (estradiol, FSH, LH, TSH, prolactin) can be drawn any time of day, but blood for testosterone levels should be drawn between 7:00 and 9:00 a.m., as this is when most men have their highest physiologic levels of blood testosterone. Men who consistently work night shifts can have blood taken for testosterone levels at their normal wake-up times. Men who inconsistently work night shifts should try to get their blood drawn for testosterone levels between 7:00 and 9:00 a.m. on a day off from work. Fasting is not required for standard fertility hormonal testing.

Repeat Testing

All blood hormone levels vary to some degree on a day-to-day basis. LH levels are known to fluctuate significantly, while FSH levels tend to show much less variation. Testosterone levels are known to vary by about 10 percent when the same person is checked multiple times on subsequent mornings.

Some clinicians recommend that if a man has a blood test showing low testosterone, then repeat blood testing should be performed to confirm this finding before starting any treatment. This is a completely valid evaluation approach. However, I typically do not get routine repeat testing for low testosterone levels. If a man is found to have an abnormally low testosterone level on one test, and on repeat testing it has moved into the normal range, then which one of those tests do I believe? Do I get a third blood test as a tiebreaker? That's a lot of baseline blood testing to do before even starting any treatments. When a man has a low baseline testosterone at initial testing, I usually assume that even if it is normal on repeat testing, that man's T levels are likely borderline at best, and he may benefit from hormonal therapy.

One thing to keep in mind is that every so often, lab errors do occur. So if an unexpected result does come back (like T levels going down after therapy has started, or blood hormone levels that do not match a man's clinical symptoms), then I recommend repeating the blood test before making definitive decisions about treatment.

Testosterone Testing Specifics

There are several different ways to determine testosterone levels. Most of the testosterone that circulates in the bloodstream is bound to proteins, the two major types being albumin and sex hormone binding globulin (SHBG). Approximately two-thirds of the testosterone in the bloodstream is bound to albumin, and about one-third is bound to SHBG. SHBG tightly binds testosterone and does not release it to be used by the cells of the body. In contrast, albumin only loosely binds to testosterone, allowing it to break free and enter into cells. About 2 percent of the testosterone in the bloodstream is unbound to any protein; this is called free testosterone. Therefore, free testosterone plus testosterone bound to albumin represents the total amount of testosterone available to the body for use in hormonal activity; this is called bioavailable testosterone.

To summarize:

Total T = (T bound to SHBG) + (T bound to albumin) + (free T)

Bioavailable T = (T bound to albumin) + (free T)

The amount of SHBG in the body varies from person to person and is affected by such factors as aging and certain disease processes. Therefore, total testosterone levels do not always accurately reflect the amount of free and bioavailable testosterone present in any particular man. Studies have shown that when only total testosterone levels are evaluated, up to 20 percent of men with true hypogonadism (i.e., low T) can be missed. Therefore, I recommend that in addition to total testosterone levels, patients should have either free testosterone level or bioavailable testosterone measured as well.

There's quite a bit of controversy in the medical literature about which test, free T or bioavailable T, is more accurate and cost-effective. My feeling is that at the present time, either test is sufficient to provide the information needed for diagnosing hypogonadism (low T).

Pricing and Insurance Codes

Blood hormone tests are often covered by insurance, but this is affected by multiple factors, including individual policy specifications and state laws on mandated fertility coverage. If fertility diagnostic tests are not covered by your insurance, non-fertility-related codes can often be used for hormone testing, since hormonal problems can have an impact on other aspects of general health besides fertility.

The codes that I have had the best success in getting insurance coverage for include:

257.2 Hypogonadism

257.9 Testicular failure

Note that after October 1, 2015, new diagnostic codes from the ICD-10 will be instituted, and codes that can be used after that time will include:

E29.1 Testicular hypogonadism

E29.9 Testicular dysfunction

What if the testing is not covered by your insurance? See Appendix C for information on pricing of fertility hormone testing without insurance coverage.

Interpretation of Hormone Testing Results

Your hormone testing report from the lab generally will show two sets of numbers: both your test result and a range of values called the reference range (typically shown to the right of your individual test finding). It is very important to remember that what's shown on the lab report as the reference range is *not* the same thing as "normal values." Rather, reference values refer to the range into which 95 percent of patients tested in a particular lab fall; this range can vary from lab to lab. The reference range often includes lab values that are well outside of the actual normal range for that hormone. For example, FSH reference ranges printed on lab reports often will be something like "1.1–15.0 mIU/mL," when in reality an FSH level over 7.0 mIU/mL is considered abnormally high. So don't use the reference ranges printed on lab reports as a definition of what is actually normal for that lab value. Instead, refer to the values indicated in this book, or discuss your results with your health care provider.

Testosterone Levels

As described previously, testosterone can be measured in three ways: total testosterone, free testosterone, and bioavailable testosterone.

For men with fertility problems, I recommend a check of total testosterone as well as either free or bioavailable testosterone. If any of these testosterone measurements are abnormal, then treatment for hypogonadism (low T) is generally recommended. See Chapter 7 for further details on the treatment of hypogonadism.

Total Testosterone (TT)

While normal total testosterone (TT) levels are 300 ng/dL or above, and ideally 500–600 ng/dL or over, there's significant controversy in the scientific and medical communities about the relationship between hypogonadism and total testosterone. The American Society of Andrology defines hypogonadism as a total testosterone level under 230 ng/dL. However, the Food and Drug Administration's definition of hypogonadism is a level of total testosterone under 300 ng/dL, and this currently seems to be the most commonly used definition in the infertility community. The problem with these definitions, however, is that the studies upon which they are based focused primarily on older males experiencing symptoms of low T, not younger men with infertility problems.

Total testosterone levels are known to decrease with age, and several studies have looked at average TT levels in different age groups. The following chart shows the result of one of these studies. The reference to "5th percentile" means that only 5 percent of the men studied had TT levels below this number, while "95th percentile" means that only 5 percent of men had TT levels over this number. The vast majority of men fall somewhere between these two figures.

Age	Average TT Level (ng/dL)	5th Percentile (ng/dL)	95th Percentile (ng/dL)
Under 25 years	692	408	956
25 to 29 years	669	388	1005
30 to 34 years	621	348	975
35 to 39 years	597	329	945
40 to 49 years	546	329	846
50 to 54 years	544	289	936
55 to 59 years	552	319	866

D. Simon, K. Nahoul, and M.-A. Charles, "Sex Hormones, Aging, Ethnicity, and Insulin Sensitivity in Men: An Overview of the TELECOM Study," in B. Oddens and A. Vermeulen, eds., *Androgens and the Aging Male* (Pantheon, 1996)

As mentioned above, most male fertility experts use 300 ng/dL as a cutoff for normal TT. However, the table shows that a man who's under fifty years old with a total testosterone of 330 ng/dL is only in the 5th percentile of men in his age group. Should such a man receive treatment for low T? This is an area of significant controversy within the male infertility community. Some experts feel that boosting T levels in men with fertility problems is likely not going to be of much clinical benefit unless the testosterone levels are very low (under 200 ng/dL). Unfortunately, there is not much good clinical data on this particular topic. Personally, I think it makes sense to attempt to get total testosterone levels to around 500–600 ng/dL to try to re-create the typical hormonal environment present in most normal men their age.

(Note: While most labs report total testosterone levels using nanograms per deciliter (ng/dL), some use a different unit of measure: picograms per microliter (pg/μL). The difference is where the decimal points are placed; for example, 3.43 pg/μL = 343 ng/dL.)

Free Testosterone (FT)

As previously described, free testosterone is the amount of testosterone that is not bound to protein in the bloodstream and can therefore freely enter the body's cells to exert its hormonal effects. Free testosterone (FT) levels can be reported in two ways. Direct testing (also called analog testing) measures the actual amount of free testosterone in the blood; normal values are 15 ng/dL or over. With a calculated FT level, total testosterone, albumin, and SHBG levels are measured and then plugged into an equation; normal calculated FT is 50 ng/dL or over.

The labs often perform the calculation themselves, but if you know your total testosterone and SHBG levels, there are free online calculators that will do this for you, such as the one on the website of the International Society for the Study of the Aging Male, www.issam.ch/freetesto.htm.

Professionals disagree about whether the direct method or the calculated method is more accurate. For clinical purposes, either the direct or the calculated FT test can be used; it's just important to note that the levels for what is considered normal are different for each. When you get back a blood test result for free T, it typically is not going to tell you whether the direct or calculated technique was used. However, if on the lab report you see results for albumin and SHBG, then you can presume that the calculated technique was used (so normal is 50 ng/dL or over). If not, then the direct technique was likely used (with normal being 15 ng/dL or over).

Bioavailable Testosterone

Bioavailable testosterone is the combination of free testosterone and the testosterone that is loosely bound to albumin. This represents the total amount of testosterone that is able to enter into the body's cells to exert their hormonal effects.

Normal bioavailable testosterone levels are 156 ng/dL or higher.

Indications for Treatment of Low T

Treatment of low testosterone is often recommended when *both* of the following criteria are fulfilled:

- Signs or symptoms of low T are present. These can include:
- Abnormal semen parameters (or abnormal sperm DNA testing)
- Sexual dysfunction problems (erectile dysfunction or ejaculatory problems)
- Symptoms of hypogonadism (see "Who Should Get Hormone Testing?" above)

and

- Abnormal results on any of the following blood tests:
- Low total testosterone: less than 500–600 ng/dL (though some fertility experts would use a cutoff of 300 mg/dL or less)
- Low free testosterone:
  - Direct/analog: less than 15 ng/dL
  - Calculated: less than 50 ng/dL
- Low bioavailable testosterone: less than 156 ng/dL

See Chapter 7 for further information on the treatment of low testosterone levels.

Luteinizing Hormone (LH)

LH, which is produced by the pituitary gland, is the hormonal signal that the brain uses to tell the testicles to make testosterone. Normal LH levels are in the range of 1.0–8.0 IU/L.

When testosterone levels decrease, the pituitary gland responds by secreting more LH, which directs the testicles to make more testosterone. But when testosterone levels are artificially high (for example, in a person taking anabolic steroids or receiving testosterone injections), then LH levels are suppressed, and testicular testosterone production decreases as a result.

When interpreting LH test results, here are some important points to remember:

- LH levels can fluctuate greatly, varying by as much as 50 percent from test to test. If testing shows unexpected results that don't match what appears to be going on, it may be a good idea to retest.
- Certain medications can have a significant impact on LH levels. Clomiphene and anastrozole (used to treat hormone irregularities) can increase LH levels, while exogenous androgens (used in androgen replacement therapy, or by men to build muscle) can decrease LH levels.

Note that HCG injections do not typically increase detectable LH levels, despite having hormonal activity similar to LH.

Interpretation of LH results is highly dependent on the accompanying total testosterone (TT) levels. For example, if LH levels are normal and TT levels are also normal, then everything's fine. But if LH levels are normal and TT is low, that suggests that the pituitary is not responding appropriately to decreased testosterone levels.

If LH is high and TT is low, that's a sign that a normal pituitary gland is responding to decreased testosterone production. If LH is high and TT is borderline or normal (300–600 ng/dL), then probably what's going on is that a testicle that was making less testosterone in the past is now responding to the increased stimulation by the extra LH in the bloodstream. But if LH is high and TT is high (over 600 ng/dL), this may signal a condition in which the body's cells don't recognize androgens (see "Androgen Insensitivity Syndrome" in Chapter 6).

When LH is low and TT is normal or high, we're seeing higher levels of androgens circulating in the bloodstream, which suppresses LH production. A common cause of this is the use of exogenous androgens for muscle building (for example, testosterone injections or use of anabolic steroids). Other, less common causes include a tumor that is secreting androgens (such as a tumor of the adrenal gland or of the testicles) or an overactive adrenal gland (see "Congenital Adrenal Hyperplasia" in Chapter 6). And a finding in which LH is low and TT is also low may indicate a problem with the pituitary gland (see "Pituitary Insufficiency (Hypopituitarism)" in Chapter 6).

Estradiol

As previously noted, estradiol is an estrogenic hormone that is normally present in all men (as well as women) and plays an important role in bone health. Recent studies suggest that low estradiol levels may also lead to symptoms of low T, including decreased energy and libido. However, estradiol levels that are too high or out of balance with total testosterone can have a potentially negative impact on male fertility (although the degree of this effect remains controversial among fertility experts) or cause other symptoms, such as male breast tissue enlargement (gynecomastia).

Normal estradiol levels in men are typically under 45 pg/mL, although if the total testosterone level is normal, I usually do not start treatment unless the estradiol level is over 59 pg/mL. (You may see different units of measurement for estradiol; for example, pg/mL or ng/dL are the same thing.)

An imbalance between estradiol and total testosterone levels can be indicated by an abnormal ratio of testosterone to estradiol, called the T/E ratio. A normal T/E ratio is 10:1 or greater. A T/E ratio of less than this can cause problems with sperm production. For example, if the total T is 510 and the estradiol is 46, then the T/E ratio is 11.1 (510 divided by 46), which is a normal level. If, however, the total T is 510 and the estradiol is 55, then the T/E ratio is 9.3 (510 divided by 55), which is too low.

For management of elevated estradiol levels or decreased T/E ratios, see Chapter 7.

Follicle-Stimulating Hormone (FSH)

FSH, as we've seen, is the chemical signal that the brain uses to tell the testicles to make sperm. FSH levels are generally considered to be normal if they're between 1.0 and 7.0 mIU/mL. In men with low sperm counts, it is important to check FSH levels to make sure that the pituitary gland is sending the correct signals to tell the testicles to make sperm.

High FSH Levels

When the sperm-producing machinery of the testicles is working well, the brain does not have to drive it very hard by producing higher FSH levels. However, when the productivity of the spermatogenic cells within the testicles starts to decrease, the brain senses this and attempts to compensate by making more FSH. This extra FSH pushes the testicles to work harder and make more sperm. Therefore, higher FSH levels typically indicate that the testicles are having a problem making sperm. In one sense, then, a high FSH is the brain's normal, healthy response to less sperm production. Therefore, when I see a man with a high FSH, the goal is not to directly decrease his FSH levels (as this excess FSH is actually helpful in trying to push the testicles to make more sperm), but rather to look for reasons why the sperm-production machinery in the testicles is not working as well as it should.

Low FSH Levels

A low FSH (under 1.0 mIU/mL) is a completely different situation, suggesting that the testicles may not be receiving the signal to tell them to make sperm. The 0.6–0.9 mIU/mL range is considered borderline; I have seen men with normal sperm production who have an FSH of 0.8 or 0.9, but levels in this range do raise the suspicion that something may be suppressing pituitary FSH production. And I get particularly concerned when FSH is 0.5 mIU/mL or less. See "Management of FSH Abnormalities" in Chapter 7.

Normal FSH Levels but Low or No Sperm

The brain has mechanisms to detect whether the testicles are producing sperm, and it uses FSH as a tool to regulate sperm production accordingly. But sometimes the pituitary does not respond appropriately to decreased sperm production by the testicles. In these cases, the pituitary is not making increased levels of FSH to drive the testicles to make more sperm. This can result in a low sperm count (oligospermia) even though the FSH level is normal. In some circumstances, treatment with clomiphene or anastrozole (which increases pituitary FSH secretion) can stimulate increased sperm production in this setting of oligospermia and normal FSH levels. See Chapter 7 for more details of hormonal treatment with clomiphene and anastrozole.

Another situation in which FSH may be normal but there's still a problem is in maturation arrest. In men with maturation arrest, the testicles may be making lots of sperm parts, but those parts are not being put together to construct whole sperm. Men with maturation arrest typically have no sperm in the ejaculate (azoospermia), as the sperm parts that are being produced cannot be seen in a semen analysis. Since the testicles are being very productive in terms of producing sperm parts, they are often of normal size, and the FSH is often normal. Essentially, the brain is tricked into thinking that everything is functioning as it should in the testicles even though the semen analysis shows no sperm. Maturation arrest can be a challenge to diagnose accurately, and it is covered more fully in Chapter 9.

Thyroid-Stimulating Hormone (TSH)

Thyroid hormone problems are an uncommon cause of male fertility problems, but they can contribute to abnormal semen parameters and sexual function in certain circumstances. The blood test for thyroid-stimulating hormone (TSH) should only be performed in men who have symptoms consistent with an underactive or overactive thyroid; see the list under "What Initial Hormone Testing Should Be Ordered?" earlier in this chapter.

The normal range for TSH is 0.4–3.0 µIU/mL. For management of low TSH (under 0.4 µIU/mL) or high TSH (over 3.0 µIU/mL), see "Management of Thyroid Abnormalities" in Chapter 7.

Inhibin B

Normal levels of inhibin B levels have not yet been completely defined. One recent study found the following ranges of inhibin B levels for three different groups of men: those with normal sperm production and those with two different types of sperm production problems.

	Inhibin (range)	FSH (for comparison)
Normal spermatogenesis	173–238 pg/mL	3.8 mIU/mL
Hypospermatogenesis	79–98 pg/mL	12.4 mIU/mL
Sertoli cell-only syndrome	18–27 pg/mL	25.9 mIU/mL

S. Grunewald, H. J. Glander, U. Paasch, and J. Kratsch, "Age-Dependent Inhibin B Concentration in Relation to FSH and Semen Sample Qualities: A Study in 2448 Men," *Reproduction* 145, no. 3 (2013): 237–44

The inhibin B test has the potential to eventually offer additional information on the state of testicular sperm production, due to its ability to directly reflect the functioning of the Sertoli cells (as opposed to indirect measures such as FSH). However, at this time, a useful role for inhibin B in the general male infertility population has not been clearly delineated, and more work needs to be performed to better define normal values. I have found that inhibin B levels can be helpful in men who have had a vasectomy and are also using exogenous androgens, in order to help determine when sperm production has started to return.

Moving Forward with the 10 Week Man Plan

Now that you've filled out the Personal Fertility Profile, had a physical examination, and had hormone testing done, I recommend that you read Chapter 5, "Recommendations for All Couples Trying to Conceive." Once you've done that, the next step is to identify which specific fertility factors may be impacting your fertility potential. Any factors in the profile for which you answered "yes" in Column 2 or 3 of the Personal Fertility Profile identifies a factor that could have a potentially negative impact on your chances of conceiving a child. Each item on the Personal Fertility Profile corresponds to an individual section in Chapter 6 or 7. These chapters will discuss each condition in depth and review possible options for managing the condition.

Once the recommended interventions have been made, most men will then have another semen analysis after ten weeks. At that point, most men should be ready to move forward with developing a Comprehensive Couple's Fertility Plan (see Chapter 8). This plan takes into account both the male and female partner's fertility factors and helps to target the most effective approaches to achieving reproductive success.

5

General Recommendations for All Couples

This chapter reviews general fertility recommendations for all couples who are trying to conceive. First are basic recommendations for men as well as information on optimizing the timing of natural intercourse. Then I review the basics of an infertility evaluation for women that can be performed either by a woman's ob-gyn or by a specialist in female fertility.

General Recommendations for All Men Trying to Conceive

A man's general health and lifestyle choices, such as exercise and a healthful diet, can play an important role in maintaining good fertility potential. Reducing the stress on the body caused by normal metabolism and toxins in the environment can help to improve the environment for healthy sperm production. Finally, the timing of intercourse can help increase a couple's chances of natural conception (for couples who are trying naturally). I'll cover all these topics in this section.

Exercise

Regular exercise can help men maintain good cardiovascular health as well as achieve and maintain a healthy weight. Of course, men with significant health problems should check with their primary care physician before starting on an exercise regimen.

The American Heart Association's current recommendations for physical activity include:

> At least 30 minutes of moderate-intensity aerobic activity a day at least five days per week (for a total of 150 minutes per week) *or* at least 25 minutes of vigorous aerobic activity at least three days per week (for a total of 75 minutes per week), *or* some combination of moderate and vigorous activity

> *and*

> Moderate- to high-intensity muscle-strengthening activity at least two days per week

Moderate aerobic activity includes brisk walking, biking at less than 10 miles per hour, ballroom dancing, doubles tennis, and gardening, among other things. Vigorous activity includes things like jogging or running, swimming laps, biking faster than 10 mph, jumping rope, and hiking uphill. Check out the American Heart Association's website, heart.org/ActivityRecommendations, for lots of useful information and suggestions about increasing your activity levels.

A few specific exercise tips for men trying to optimize their fertility potential:

- *Avoid tight biking-style shorts.* One of the primary ways the body regulates its temperature is for the scrotum to relax and increase its surface area, which promotes evaporation of sweat. Very tight workout pants prevent this scrotal relaxation and can result in increased scrotal temperatures, which can have a negative impact on sperm production.

- *Avoid excessive bicycle riding.* The combination of the riding position, narrow biking seat, and tight biking shorts all combine to produce a negative environment for sperm quality. I recommend that patients avoid biking more than fifty miles per week if they are actively trying to conceive a child. Shorter bike rides (less than fifty miles per week) are not likely to make much of a difference, especially if you don't wear tight biking shorts.

Can Too Much Exercise Be Bad for Sperm Production?

Studies have shown that too much exercise may be detrimental to sperm quality in some men. While individuals vary greatly, men who exercised for one hour three times a week have been shown to have better semen parameters than elite triathletes undergoing intensive daily training for Ironman-type competitions. Though changes were also seen in sperm counts and motility, the most dramatic effects were seen on sperm morphology. One factor to keep in mind is that the elite triathletes were putting in over two hundred miles of biking per week as part of their training, and this amount of biking by itself is known to be bad for sperm production. However, other types of intensive activity, such as running more than sixty miles a week, have also been associated with significant decreases in semen parameters in some men. Studies of marathon runners show that while most had normal semen parameters, about 10 percent were found to have elevated levels of semen abnormalities while they were training.

It's been suggested that overtraining reduces sperm quality by increasing oxidative stress (see "Antioxidants" later in this chapter for more information) and raising scrotal temperature. Every person's individual exercise threshold is going to be different, but if you've got abnormal semen parameters and are having trouble conceiving, and if you're working out intensively, I recommend moderating your exercise routine.

Dietary Recommendations

Multiple studies have shown an association between a healthful, well-balanced diet and improved semen parameters. There is no one set "male fertility diet"; rather, there are general guidelines about foods that have been found to be either helpful or detrimental to optimal sperm production. The goal is to make dietary changes that are sustainable. If you try to make changes that are too radical to maintain, chances are that you're not going to stick to them, and so you won't see any real improvements in fertility potential—plus you might stress yourself out in the process. The guidelines I present here are designed to encourage overall better dietary choices without being too strict to maintain.

Good Foods for Male Fertility

In general, aim for a well-balanced diet, with a focus on these healthful foods:

- *Fresh fruits and vegetables.* Try to get at least five to six servings per day. Green leafy vegetables are an especially good natural source of beneficial folic acid. If you can find and afford organic produce, it will reduce your exposure to pesticide residues.

- *Lean protein in moderate amounts.* Good choices include fish (but stay away from types that are often high in mercury, including swordfish, king mackerel, shark, and tilefish), skinless chicken and turkey, legumes (beans, lentils, peas), nuts (including nut butters) and seeds, egg whites, low-fat dairy (skim or 1 percent milk, low-fat cheeses such as cottage cheese, feta, Camembert, and ricotta), and oatmeal.

- *Complex carbohydrates.* While carbs have gotten something of a bad rap lately, studies have shown that some intake of carbohydrates may be important for maintaining good sperm production. Whole, unprocessed carbohydrates provide energy, nutrients, and fiber and don't spike your blood sugar the way highly processed carbs do. Instead of white bread and pasta, look for whole-grain types. Go for rolled or steel-cut oats instead of instant oatmeal (which is often high in sugar, too). Try different whole grains such barley, quinoa, brown rice, or wild rice. Pick sweet potatoes, corn, lima or butter beans, peas, lentils, and other types of beans instead of white potatoes. And, of course, fruits and non-starchy vegetables provide carbohydrates as well as other nutrients.

- *Unsaturated fats.* These can help lower LDL (bad) cholesterol, and some can improve levels of HDL (good) cholesterol. Unsaturated fats come from plants and fish sources and are liquid at room temperature. Good sources of this type of fat include oily fish (such as salmon, tuna, herring, sardines, and anchovies), vegetable and seed oils (such as olive, canola, peanut, flaxseed, safflower, and sunflower), nuts (for example, pecans, almonds, and hazelnuts), and seeds (including sesame, pumpkin, and sunflower).

The Bad Fats

Some fat in the diet is necessary for health, but make sure you're eating more of the healthful types of fats mentioned above, and less of these problematic fats:

- *Saturated fats.* These come largely from animal products, such as high-fat dairy products (butter, cream, ice cream, whole milk), high-fat cheeses (cheddar, Swiss, Gouda, Parmesan, Gruyere, cream cheese), fatty cuts of meat (including bacon and lard), and poultry skin. But they can also be found in some plant sources, such as palm and coconut oils. If the fat is solid at room temperature, then it's saturated.

- *Red meat.* If you eat red meat, limit your intake to about 18 ounces per week, and go for leaner cuts of beef (such as eye

round, sirloin tip, top round, bottom round, and top sirloin)
and pork (such as loin and tenderloin).

- *Fried foods.* They often contain unhealthful fats, plus lots of
  calories.

- *Trans fats.* Avoid these, which are vegetable oils that have
  undergone an industrial process to solidify them and extend
  their shelf life. They've been shown to raise LDL (bad) cholesterol and lower HDL (good) cholesterol—exactly the
  opposite of what you want. They're often found in processed baked goods (cookies, pie crusts, cakes, pizza dough,
  hamburger buns), snack foods (crackers, chips, cookies,
  candy, prepackaged popcorn), fried foods, frozen dinners,
  and some types of margarine. Food producers are required
  by law to list trans fats on a product's Nutrition Facts label,
  and you can also check the ingredients list for the words
  "hydrogenated" and "partially hydrogenated," which tell
  you that the product contains trans fats.

Is Soy a Problem?

Soy products—tofu, edamame, soy sauce, soy milk, soy flour—
contain phytoestrogens, substances with known estrogenic (female
hormonal) activity. Several studies have shown a possible link
between regular soy product consumption and decreased semen
parameters. Although these findings are controversial, I recommend that men avoid regular soy intake while trying to impregnate
their partner.

Sugar: It's Not So Sweet

Simple sugars spike blood glucose levels and offer lots of calories
with little nutrition. I suggest you avoid them when possible. In
addition to the obvious suspects, such as sweetened drinks (sugary
soda, sweetened tea, fruit juice), candy, cookies, cake, and jams and

jellies, you might be surprised by the sugar content in ketchup, sauces, and dressings. Read labels and look for the various names that sugar hides under: sucrose, glucose, fructose, lactose, maltose, raw (or brown or beet) sugar, molasses, evaporated cane juice, cane sugar, maple sugar or syrup, high fructose corn syrup, and turbinado sugar.

Extreme Diets for Weight Loss

Extreme diets that eliminate whole categories of foods are generally not good for fertility. If you want to lose weight, see "Weight Loss and Maintenance" in Chapter 6 for more information on effective weight loss strategies that can also have fertility benefits.

Antioxidants

What Is Oxidative Stress?

The body's normal metabolic processes create by-products called reactive oxygen species (ROS), also called free radicals. These metabolic by-products have the potential to negatively affect individual cells, tissues, and organs, but under normal circumstances the body is well equipped with antioxidants, substances that mop up excess reactive oxygen species before significant problems occur. Small amounts of ROS are normally present within the genital duct system, and in fact they are thought to play an important positive role in normal sperm production and function.

However, when the amount of ROS becomes greater than the body's normal cleanup mechanisms can easily handle, the result is increased oxidative stress on the body. Unfortunately, sperm are especially sensitive to oxidative stress, which can result in cellular and DNA damage and lead to decreases in both sperm numbers and quality.

Causes of Oxidative Stress

One reason for increased levels of ROS in the genital duct system is the presence of higher-than-normal levels of white blood cells, which can be a sign of infection or inflammation. As mentioned in Chapter 3, *pyospermia* is the term for semen that contains elevated levels of WBCs. The presence of immature sperm cells may be another cause of oxidative stress. Increased scrotal temperature and varicoceles can also play a role in oxidative stress.

Certain lifestyle factors increase oxidative stress. These include:

- Use of cigarettes or other tobacco products, or exposure to secondhand smoke
- Exposure to chemicals or environmental toxins
- Excessive alcohol intake
- Use of marijuana or other drugs

Management of Oxidative Stress

Managing oxidative stress in men generally takes two approaches: eliminating oxidative stress factors where possible, and supplementing with antioxidants.

Chapter 6 discusses ways to decrease or eliminate risk factors for elevated oxidative stress, such as treatment of pyospermia, treatment of varicoceles, and reducing scrotal temperature. I also strongly recommend that you reduce oxidative stress by stopping smoking, avoiding drug use, reducing alcohol intake, and reducing or eliminating exposure to chemicals and environmental toxins that may be producing excessive amounts of ROS.

Over-the-counter antioxidant supplements can help to clean up ROS within the genital duct system. While different male fertility experts take different approaches to antioxidant therapies—some reserve this for men who have certain significant risk factors (such as tobacco use or pyospermia), and other clinicians only use antioxidants if elevated levels of oxidative stress are found upon testing (see the box "Oxidative Stress Adduct Test")—my personal preference is to start all of my fertility patients on antioxidant therapy. The goal of managing male factor fertility is to optimize the environment for sperm production as much as possible, and oxidative stress impacts a significant number of these men. Over-the-counter antioxidant supplements are easy to obtain, are inexpensive, and have minimal associated risks and side effects, so I generally suggest that patients continue using these supplements until pregnancy is achieved with their partner. I'll discuss the different types of supplements below.

Oxidative Stress Adduct Test

A specialized test, called the oxidative stress adduct (OSA) test, can directly measure the degree of oxidative damage to the sperm. OSA testing is available from Reprosource (www.reprosource.com) and is part of the company's Advanced Semen Report, which also includes DNA fragmentation index testing. See Chapter 11 for more detailed information on OSA testing.

Antioxidant Supplements

A quick search of the Internet will turn up a bewildering array of nonprescription supplements designed to boost male fertility: ProXeed Plus, Fertility Blend for Men, FertilAid, Motility Boost, Count Boost, Ultra Fertile Plus, Coast Male Fertility Supplement, and Conception XR, to name just a few. In general, though, most of these supplements contain some mixture of the following common nutrients:

Vitamin A

Vitamin C

Vitamin E

Selenium

Zinc

L-carnitine

Acetyl-L-carnitine

Coenzyme Q10

Folic acid

Other ingredients you may see in these supplements include vitamin B_6, vitamin B_{12}, vitamin D, vitamin K, copper, manganese, fructose, arginine, quercetin, L-glutathione, niacin, thiamine, riboflavin, iodine, and chromium.

Some supplements say they contain "proprietary blends" of ingredients, which can include herbs such as maca root, Asian ginseng, and various seed extracts. "Medications and Supplements" in Chapter 6 has more information on herbal supplements.

The cost of these commercially available supplements varies significantly—they can cost anywhere from $20 to $125 a month, or even more.

I currently do not use any of the commercially available name-brand male fertility supplements in my practice. This is not because I question their efficacy, but rather because I have not seen any convincing data that these commercial formulations offer any additional benefit over generic supplements that cost significantly less. One potential benefit of the commercial supplements, however, may be convenience: they often combine multiple ingredients in a single pill, thus decreasing the number of pills that need to be taken daily. Still, that convenience comes at a price.

Most studies that look at the effects of antioxidants and over-the-counter supplements on male fertility have been small or not placebo-controlled, and thus their results must be taken with a healthy degree of skepticism. Even so, I think the existing data on the effects of antioxidants on semen parameters and IVF outcomes provide good enough evidence to advocate the use of the following four supplements.

- *Coenzyme Q10 (CoQ10).* Also known as ubiquinone or ubiquinol, CoQ10 is a vitamin-like substance that has antioxidant properties and is also involved in cellular energy production. Studies have associated CoQ10 supplementation with improvements in semen parameters, though the literature has not to date documented a definitive improvement in pregnancy rates.
- *L-carnitine.* L-carnitine is an amino acid (a building block for proteins) that has antioxidant properties and is also involved in cellular fatty acid metabolism. Supplementation of L-carnitine has been associated with improvement in semen parameters (especially motility).

L-Carnitine and Cardiovascular Risk

Recent research from the Cleveland Clinic has linked L-carnitine intake to increased cardiovascular risk factors, alongside fat and cholesterol. L-carnitine is found in high levels in red meat. When consumed by people who regularly eat red meat, L-carnitine can be broken down by intestinal bacteria into TMAO, a by-product that can lead to increased atherosclerotic vessel damage. Interestingly, vegetarians may not have the necessary bacteria in their intestines to break down L-carnitine into TMAO. More research is certainly needed on this topic. My current take on the subject is this: L-carnitine may modestly increase cardiovascular risk if taken over long periods of time. I therefore only recommend that men take L-carnitine while they are trying to achieve a pregnancy. Once their partner is pregnant, I recommend that they stop all fertility-related supplements. Men who have a strong personal or family history of cardiovascular disease should discuss L-carnitine use with their cardiologist or primary care physician before starting this supplement.

- *Folic acid.* Folic acid (vitamin B9) is a vitamin found in a variety of foods, including green leafy vegetables. Folic acid supplementation is strongly recommended in all women wishing to become pregnant due to its proven ability to reduce the risk of neural tube defects in newborns. In men, there is some evidence that folate deficiency can lead to decreased fertility, as well as an increased risk of birth defects.

Suggested Antioxidant Regimen

I suggest that my patients take the following over-the-counter supplements while trying to conceive:

1. A general antioxidant formula containing the following vitamins and minerals, once a day:
   - Vitamin A: 10,000 IU
   - Vitamin C: 250 mg
   - Vitamin E: 200 IU
   - Selenium: 15 mcg
   - Zinc: 7.5 mcg
2. L-carnitine: 500 mg once a day (or 1,000 mg every other day)
3. Coenzyme Q10 (CoQ10): 200 mg once a day (or 400 mg every other day)
4. Folic acid: 400 mcg once a day (or 800 mcg every other day)

The cheapest brand that I have found so far for these antioxidants is Spring Valley, which typically can be found in Walmart stores (with the antioxidant under the name "Antioxidant with Minerals"). Similar brands are often stocked at chain drugstores such as Walgreens and supermarkets such as Kroger, but may be more expensive. If you can't find them in a store near you, you can order them online. Together these four supplements currently cost about $15–20 a month at Walmart or Walmart.com.

I typically recommend stopping other multivitamins or supplements (such as fish oil) while taking this regimen. Some nutrients, such as vitamin E, are fat soluble and can potentially reach toxic levels within the body if taken in too large a quantity. There are also some concerns about an increased risk of prostate cancer with vitamin E levels that exceed 400 IU per day. Other supplements that can be beneficial at low doses, such as zinc, can have a negative impact on sperm production when taken at higher levels.

Once a pregnancy has been established, the supplements should be discontinued.

Optimizing Natural Intercourse

This section is for couples who are working on trying to achieve a pregnancy naturally through timed intercourse.

The Fertile Window

The most fertile time in a women's menstrual cycle is generally the six days prior to and including the day of ovulation (called the "fertile window"), though the length of this window may vary somewhat from woman to woman. The last two days just prior to ovulation are the times of highest fertility during this window. Intercourse at other times outside of this six-day window are less likely to result in a pregnancy, although conception can still occur in some circumstances.

Studies have shown that frequent intercourse, every one to two days, during the fertile window results in the highest pregnancy rates. No significant difference in pregnancy rates has been shown in studies comparing intercourse every day with intercourse every other day. The American Society of Reproductive Medicine therefore recommends that natural fertility can be maximized in most couples with regular intercourse (every one to two days) beginning after the woman's menstrual flow has stopped and continuing through the time of ovulation (see the next section for how to predict ovulation).

However, a strict regimen of timed intercourse can cause significant stress and relationship strain in some couples. If this is a factor for you, know that a slightly decreased rate of intercourse during this time—two to three times per week—yields nearly equivalent rates of pregnancy.

Methods of Predicting Ovulation

Counting Backward from the Start of Menstruation

Day 1 of the menstrual cycle, which is the first day of full menstrual flow, typically occurs fourteen days after ovulation. If a woman's cycles are very regular, this can be used to help predict the next month's day of ovulation.

Basal Body Temperature

Starting approximately two days after ovulation, there is a sustained temperature increase of about 1°F that can be detected when the woman measures her body temperature each morning before rising. If a woman's cycles are very regular, then charting basal body temperature can help predict ovulation.

Cervical Mucus

The cervical mucus typically becomes slippery and clear and increases in volume around the time of ovulation, starting to increase about five or six days before ovulation and peaking within two or three days of ovulation. Women can check the consistency of their cervical mucus by examining the discharge from the vagina or inserting a clean finger into the vagina. However, ovulation can occur without obvious cervical mucus changes.

Physical Symptoms

In many women, physical symptoms such as headaches, breast tenderness, mood swings, or changes in libido occur approximately seven to ten days prior to the menstrual period. Mittelschmerz, which is lower abdominal or pelvic pain on one side, is associated with ovulation in some women. However, determining ovulation on the basis of these symptoms is typically accurate only about half of the time.

Ovulation Detection Kits

Ovulation detection kits that measure luteinizing hormone (LH) in a woman's urine can be obtained at drugstores without a prescription. A woman tests her urine every day with one of the strips included in the kit. When the urinary LH reaches a certain level (called LH surge), the test strip changes color. Ovulation typically occurs within two days of the LH surge. Clear Plan Easy and OvuKit One-Step are two good brands that are widely available. Be aware, though, that even with a good-quality kit, there is about a 7 percent false positive rate per cycle, with the kit incorrectly identifying the day of ovulation.

Follow the instructions on whichever kit you have purchased. Most recommend starting testing seventeen to eighteen days prior to the predicted first day of the woman's period. For example, for a woman with a twenty-eight-day cycle, testing could begin on day 10 or 11. Generally, it is best to do the test between 10:00 a.m. and 2:00 p.m. unless the directions specify otherwise. Once the color change is seen, it is not necessary to check further during that cycle.

If your partner is taking clomiphene (Clomid), the ovulation detection kits can still be used, though with some modifications. The kit can provide inaccurate results if it's used on the days when she is actively taking the clomiphene.

- A woman taking clomiphene on days 3 through 7 of her cycle should start checking for an LH surge on day 10.
- A woman taking clomiphene on days 5 through 9 of her cycle should start checking for an LH surge on day 12.

For further information about using an ovulation detection kit if a woman is taking clomiphene, see the gynecologist or infertility specialist who prescribed the medication.

Position During Intercourse

There are plenty of theories out there about how to increase your chances of natural conception with particular positions and techniques, such as having the woman remain lying on her back for a period of time following intercourse. Some also say that you can improve your chances of having a boy or a girl depending on the position you use. The American Society of Reproductive Medicine has reviewed the available data and found that technique and position during intercourse do *not* make a difference in terms of either improved fertility or the chances of having a boy or girl. And women do not need to stay on their backs following ejaculation, as studies have shown that sperm are present within the cervical channels within seconds of ejaculation.

Fertility Evaluation for Women

An integrated fertility plan that takes into account both male and female issues offers couples the best chance of establishing a pregnancy. While this book offers the latest guidelines for evaluating and managing male fertility problems, it is important to keep in mind what is going on from the female side as well. I always recommend that couples going through the 10 Week Man Plan also make sure that the woman is undergoing an evaluation during this period, if she has not done so already.

There are some exceptions, such as couples in which the man has no sperm at all (azoospermia) and the woman decides to put her evaluation on hold until the cause of her partner's issue can be determined. This is a reasonable approach. However, for the majority of couples, a simultaneous evaluation of both the male and female sides is the best approach.

Women often have their initial fertility evaluation with their regular ob-gyn, the doctor they see for their routine Pap smears and other general gynecologic issues. Most ob-gyns have been trained to perform a basic female fertility evaluation and may offer basic treatments such as clomiphene. If these initial efforts are not successful, then the woman is usually referred to a fertility specialist.

Specialists in female fertility are called reproductive endocrinologists, or REs. REs generally see only fertility patients, and most do not deliver babies; they will pass the woman back to her regular ob-gyn once she is eight to ten weeks pregnant.

At the initial appointment, the RE looks over the woman's history, performs a physical exam, and reviews the results of whatever previous fertility testing has already been performed. On the basis of this assessment, he or she will determine if further testing is indicated. The fertility evaluation checks to see whether the woman is ovulating normally, whether she has any hormone abnormalities, and whether there are any structural problems (such as with the fallopian tubes or the uterus) that may be contributing to an inability to conceive.

Besides treating any potentially reversible problems that are diagnosed, REs offer a variety of treatments that can be used to increase the chances of pregnancy for a couple. See Appendix D for more information.

Basic Female Fertility Evaluation

Basic fertility testing for a woman includes:

1. Basic fertility history
   - Prior pregnancy history
   - Abnormal cycle length (less than 27 days or greater than 32 days)
   - History or symptoms of endometriosis
   - History of cervical procedures (such as LEEP for cervical dysplasia)
   - Known tubal or uterine problems
   - Family history of known female fertility problems
   - Prior history of surgery involving any of the reproductive organs

2. Blood hormone testing
   - Day 21 progesterone: 3 ng/mL or greater is consistent with ovulation, while over 10 ng/mL increases the likelihood of conception
   - Thyroid hormone level
   - Prolactin
   - Estradiol

3. Ovarian reserve testing
   - Day 3 FSH: normal is under 10 IU/L, abnormal is over 15 IU/L
   - Antral follicle count by transvaginal ultrasound, performed within the first four days of the cycle: 5 or more follicles is good, 2–4 follicles is fair, 1–2 follicles is poor
   - Clomiphene challenge test, with FSH levels checked on day 3 of the cycle, clomiphene taken on days 5 through 9, and the FSH level repeated on day 10: normal FSH on

day 3 is less than 10 IU/L, while on day 10 it should be less than 3 IU/L; an abnormal FSH level on either day would be more than 15 IU/L

4. Transvaginal ultrasound
    - Can be used to do an antral follicle count (see above)
    - Also used to evaluate for pelvic masses, ovarian cysts, fibroids, and structural uterine abnormalities

5. Hysterosalpingogram, an imaging test that can look for structural abnormalities of the uterus and fallopian tubes

6. Sonohysterogram, which uses ultrasound to check for abnormalities of the uterus and uterine lining

7. Laparoscopy, an outpatient procedure in which a small, lighted scope is used to look into the abdomen under anesthesia, checking for problems such as endometriosis, ovarian cysts, and scar tissue

Not all of these tests are indicated for every woman. Testing should be individualized for each patient depending upon her personal history and clinical situation.

Common Female Fertility Problems

Ovulatory Dysfunction

Women with ovulatory dysfunction may be releasing an egg at only irregular intervals or not at all. A variety of treatments are available for women with ovulatory dysfunction. Some treatments are aimed at the source of the problem, such as metformin in women with polycystic ovarian syndrome. Medications such as clomiphene, tamoxifen, and letrozole can often normalize abnormal ovulation. Ovulation can also be triggered with an injection of HCG given at the correct time in a woman's cycle. Gonadotropins can also be used to overcome ovulatory problems.

Polycystic Ovarian Syndrome (PCOS)

Women with PCOS produce too many androgens (male hormones), which can interfere with ovulation. Obesity is a significant risk factor for PCOS, but women who are not obese can have this hormonal problem as well. Treatments include exercise and weight loss for women in whom obesity is contributing to their hormone imbalance. Medications such as metformin are often used to decrease insulin resistance and help to normalize ovulation. If these are not effective, then hormonal medications such as clomiphene, tamoxifen, or letrozole are often helpful in reestablishing normal ovulation. A more aggressive treatment option involves making small holes in the ovaries; these holes reduce the amount of ovarian tissue present, which helps alleviate the hormonal problems.

Endometriosis

Abnormal deposits of endometrial tissue can cause blockage of the fallopian tubes, as well as interfere with the transfer of eggs from the ovaries to the fallopian tubes. Endometriosis is often painful, but sometimes there are no symptoms at all. One type of treatment involves prescribing medications that suppress hormone production, but a pregnancy cannot be established while these medications are being taken. The diagnosis of endometriosis is generally made by laparoscopy, and definitive treatment is typically achieved by laparoscopic ablation (destroying the abnormal tissue in a laparascopic procedure).

Pelvic Adhesions

Scar tissue can be present within the pelvis as a result of prior surgeries, infections, or endometriosis. Known as adhesions, this scar tissue can cause fallopian tube obstructions or interfere with the transfer of eggs from the ovaries to the fallopian tubes. Adhesions can be treated laparoscopically, but the scar tissue may come back over time.

Uterine Abnormalities

Abnormalities of the structure of the uterus, such as a uterine septum (congenital malformation), polyps (spots of abnormal endometrial tissue growth), and fibroids (abnormal growths of muscle tissue), can make it difficult to establish or maintain a pregnancy. Some of these uterine problems can be managed with a minimally invasive procedure called a hysteroscopy. However, larger fibroids or more severe structural abnormalities may require laparoscopic or open surgical repair.

Ovarian Cysts

An ovarian cyst is a fluid-filled sac or pocket on the ovary. Many ovarian cysts come and go, and do not cause fertility problems. However, if ovarian cysts get large enough, they can interfere with normal ovulation, or even cause obstructive problems. Large cysts can be treated laparoscopically or sometimes aspirated (drained).

Decreased Ovulatory Reserve or Premature Ovarian Failure

A woman is born with all of the eggs she will ever have. Menopause is reached when the reserve of eggs has been exhausted. Decreased ovulatory reserve, or a low egg supply, is more common in women over the age of forty, but it is sometimes seen in woman as young as their late twenties. Normal ovulatory cycles become less common when the egg supply is low, and these women do not respond as well to fertility medications such as gonadotropins. Premature ovarian failure is defined as the onset of menopause before the age of forty.

6

Optimizing Reversible Male-Factor Issues

This chapter is a review of a wide array of factors that can contribute to male infertility. As described earlier, this chapter is not designed to be read from start to finish. In order to save time and effort on your part, only those areas to which you answered yes on the Personal Fertility Profile should be reviewed. This strategy will provide you with a personalized and time-efficient management plan for optimizing male fertility parameters.

The first eight sections of the Personal Fertility Profile are covered in this chapter. Abnormalities found in Section 9 of the profile (Review of Hormone Testing) are addressed in Chapter 7.

Reversible Semen Parameter Factors

Section 1 of the Personal Fertility Profile reviews potentially reversible male-factor problems that can be uncovered with a careful review of the semen analysis results: low ejaculate volume, acidic semen pH or fructose negative, abnormal viscosity or liquefaction, pyospermia, and clumping of sperm.

Abnormal Ejaculate Volume

Most labs report a normal ejaculate volume as above 1.0 cc to 2.0 cc, and the 2010 WHO guidelines use 1.5 cc as the lower limit of normal). I personally use 1.0 cc as the cutoff level for normal, although men with persistently borderline volumes (around 1.0 cc) should probably be checked for problems such as retrograde ejaculation. Usually, however, when I see a patient with a border-line ejaculate volume, it is later found to be normal upon repeat testing after a sufficient period of abstinence (see below).

Labs often report an upper limit on normal volume (for example, 6.0 cc), but I am not usually concerned about ejaculate volumes higher than this. If I see an ejaculate volume that is very high (for example, 20 cc) in someone with a neurologic disorder or someone with prior urethral surgery, then I get suspicious that the ejaculate may contain some urine that is leaking out with the ejaculate (in which case the pH should be acidic, reflecting that acidity of the urine). This is a rare finding, though, and high ejaculate volumes are typically fine, just representing a more robust production of fluid volume by the prostate and seminal vesicles.

A more worrisome finding is to have a low ejaculate volume, less than 1.0 cc. The most common reason for a low ejaculate volume is a failure to collect the entire specimen in the collection cup. It is always important to let the lab know if you have missed part of your ejaculate collection (as well as a rough estimate of what percentage of the specimen was lost) so that this can be taken into consideration during review of the test results.

If none of the specimen was missed on collection, then the most common reasons for a low ejaculate volume include:

- *Short abstinence interval.* Before providing a specimen for semen analysis, you should abstain from sexual activity of any kind, including masturbation, for two to five days. If you abstain for less than two days, the seminal vesicles may not have time to fully recharge, and this can contribute to a lower than normal ejaculate volume.

- *Retrograde ejaculation.* This is a situation where the bladder neck does not tighten down as it should during ejaculation, and either all or part of the ejaculate flows backward into the bladder. See "Retrograde Ejaculation" later in this chapter for more details.

- *Low testosterone levels.* The functions of the seminal vesicles and prostate gland are influenced by testosterone levels. Low testosterone levels can lead to a decrease in ejaculate volume in some men.

- *Ejaculatory dysfunction.* This occurs when the muscular vas deferens does not properly transport the sperm from the epididymis to the urethra. A severe form of this, in which no fluid comes into the urethra at all, is called anejaculation. Common reasons for ejaculatory dysfunction include neurologic problems (such as spinal cord injury or diabetes mellitus) and certain medications (such as antidepressants). See "Ejaculatory Problems" later in this chapter for more information.

- *Seminal vasculopathy.* The seminal vesicles can become dysfunctional and fail to contract, leading to decreased amounts of seminal vesicle fluid entering into the ejaculate. Neurologic problems, such as diabetes mellitus, are the most common cause of seminal vasculopathy.

- *Ejaculatory duct obstruction (EDO).* In men with EDO, the fluid from the vas deferens and seminal vesicles is blocked from entering the urethra. This can be either a partial or complete blockage. See "Ejaculatory Problems" later in this chapter for further information on EDO.

- *Dehydration.* If a man is very dehydrated at the time of specimen collection, it can potentially play a role in decreased ejaculate volumes, although this has not been studied extensively. For men with a borderline ejaculate volume, I recommend that they come in well hydrated for any follow-up semen analysis testing, drinking enough fluids to keep the urine pale yellow (generally a good sign of adequate hydration).

Acidic Semen pH or Fructose Negative

As described in Chapter 3, the pH of the ejaculate is normally alkaline, with a pH of 7.5 or higher (the seminal vesicles produce a large volume of alkaline fluid, substantially more than the acidic fluid produced by the prostate). The seminal vesicles also produce fructose. So when the ejaculate has an alkaline pH and contains fructose, then fluid from the seminal vesicles is successfully entering the ejaculate.

The ejaculatory ducts carry the fluid from the vas deferens and seminal vesicles to the urethra, where it is joined by the prostatic fluid. Complete blockage of the ejaculatory ducts blocks all fluids coming from the testicles and seminal vesicles, so that only fluid from the prostate enters into the ejaculate. (See "Ejaculatory Problems" later in this chapter for more information on ejaculatory duct obstruction.) Therefore men with complete ejaculatory duct blockage typically have no sperm at all in the ejaculate (azoospermia), low ejaculate volume (less than 1.0 cc), acidic semen pH (under 7.5) and no fructose in the semen.

Other potential causes for abnormalities in semen pH and fructose include:

- *Lab error.* Because of this possibility, when the results of the semen analysis don't match up with what seems to be going on in the man's body, I recommend repeat testing to rule out a simple error.

- *Incomplete collection.* The last part of the semen that is ejaculated contains most of the seminal vesicle fluid. So if the last part of the specimen wasn't collected in the container, the results could come back as abnormal.

- *Seminal vesicle inflammation.* This usually causes elevated levels of semen white blood cells.

Of note, many fertility experts feel that semen fructose testing should never really be needed, since low volume, a complete lack of sperm, and an acidic pH should be enough to clearly indicate the presence of ejaculatory duct blockage or absence.

Abnormal Semen Liquefaction and Viscosity

The fluid from the seminal vesicles causes sperm to stick together, or coagulate, in order to hold the sperm near the cervical opening and protect them from the harsh vaginal environment. The enzymes in the prostatic fluid then cause the semen to gradually liquefy, thereby allowing the sperm to enter the cervical canal. The rate at which the semen liquefies is often measured as viscosity (with a normal result being under 2) or liquefaction time (with normal ranging between 5 and 25 minutes).

Sometimes a semen analysis will show a prolonged liquefaction time (more than 30 minutes) or abnormal viscosity (over 2). In most circumstances, a repeat analysis—especially one performed at a fertility-specific lab—will show normal results, so nothing further needs to be done. However, a persistently abnormal finding could signify one of the following problems:

- *Dehydration.* Dehydration can lead to increased semen viscosity. As noted above, I recommend repeat testing with attention to proper hydration beforehand. A good goal is to drink enough to keep the urine pale yellow.

- *Infection or inflammation.* In some circumstances, infection or inflammation of the genital duct (especially of the prostate) can increase semen viscosity. High levels of white blood cells (pyospermia) are typically present if there is an active infection or inflammation. See below for more details on pyospermia.

- *Improper semen collection.* Most of the prostate fluid is in the first third of the ejaculate, while the seminal vesicle fluid is generally in the last part of the specimen. If part of the collection is missed, this can have an impact on the coagulation and liquefaction of the specimen, depending on which part was lost.

Persistent high sperm viscosity or elevated liquefaction times are rare in the absence of dehydration or infection, but where either is a problem, it can be generally be overcome with sperm washing combined with intrauterine insemination (see Appendix D). If questions arise concerning the fertility impact of abnormal semen liquefaction, post-coital testing can be done to see if sperm are efficiently making it into the cervical canal (see "Post-Coital Testing" in Chapter 11).

Elevated White Blood Cells (Pyospermia)

Pyospermia, or an elevated number of white blood cells (WBCs) in the semen, signifies the presence of inflammation within the male genital duct system. The laboratory diagnosis of pyospermia can be difficult, since immature sperm cells look very similar to WBCs in a semen specimen. "White Blood Cells or Round Cells" in Chapter 3 provides details on how to distinguish whether elevated numbers of so-called round cells in the semen actually represent the presence of pyospermia.

While an increased number of immature sperm cells generally is not considered to be clinically significant, inflammation in the genital duct system can have a significant negative impact on the fertility potential of some men. Inflammation can be due to either an infection (bacterial, viral, fungal) or to a non-infectious cause (for example, nonspecific inflammation of the prostate or epididymis). Only about 20 percent of genital duct inflammation seen in male infertility patients is due to an infection.

Fertility Impact of Pyospermia

A normal by-product of the body's metabolic processes is reactive oxygen species (ROS), also called free radicals (see "What Is Oxidative Stress?" in Chapter 5). Under normal circumstances the body is very well equipped to mop up these ROS before they can cause any damage to cells, tissues, or organs. Small amounts of ROS are produced by the sperm themselves, but white blood cells generate very large amounts of these damaging substances. In pyospermia, with its elevated levels of white blood cells, the increased amounts of ROS can overwhelm the body's cleanup mechanisms, resulting in oxidative stress. Sperm are especially sensitive to oxidative stress-related damage because of the compact structure of their DNA (genetic material), their natural lack of antioxidants, and their inability to effectively repair damage.

Pyospermia has been associated with an increased risk of several male reproductive problems, including:

- Decreased sperm density, motility, and morphology
- Elevated levels of sperm DNA fragmentation
- Decreased pregnancy rates and poor embryo progression with IVF

- Inflammation-related formation of anti-sperm antibodies

Evaluation of Pyospermia

Clinically significant pyospermia is typically considered to be a white blood cell count over 1 million per cc *or* a WBC count of over 10–15 per high power field (hpf) (different labs use different methods for counting WBCs).

It is important to distinguish between asymptomatic pyospermia and symptomatic pyospermia. In asymptomatic pyospermia, a man's semen analysis shows elevated WBC, but he has no symptoms. Men with symptomatic pyospermia have elevated levels of semen WBCs in addition to symptoms of inflammation, which can include:

- Discomfort in the scrotal area or in the perineum (the region behind the scrotum where the prostate gland sits)
- Urinary symptoms, such as burning with urination, needing to urinate frequently, discomfort with urination, or cloudy foul-smelling urine
- Urethral discharge (discolored fluid draining from the end of the penis)

In patients coming in for fertility-related reasons, asymptomatic pyospermia is much more common than symptomatic pyospermia. If there are symptoms associated with the elevated WBC count, then the risk of an active infection is significantly increased, and urine testing is indicated. Possible tests include a urinalysis, a urine culture, or screening for chlamydia and gonorrhea (STDs typically can be diagnosed by testing the urine, but sometimes a urethral swab is needed).

Diagnostic codes that can be used for these tests include:

Diagnosis	ICD-9 code (before Oct. 2015)	ICD-10 (Oct. 2015 and later)
Acute cystitis	600.11	N30.0
Chronic cystitis	V70.0	N30.2
Prostatitis	601.1	N41.9
STD screening	V74.5	Z11.3

Treatment of Pyospermia

Asymptomatic Pyospermia

As mentioned above, most men being evaluated for fertility who are found to have elevated levels of WBCs in their semen have asymptomatic pyospermia. In about 80 percent of these cases, the pyospermia is from non-infectious causes, meaning that somewhere in the genital duct system (most commonly the prostate) there is some inflammation not caused by an infection. Asymptomatic prostatitis, or prostate inflammation, is fairly common; usually no cause can be found.

Because most men with pyospermia do not have an infection, some fertility specialists choose not to treat them with antibiotics, and instead rely only on only anti-inflammatory medications to clear the WBCs from the genital tract. I would not want to miss the 20 percent of men whose pyospermia is the result of an infection, and so I usually treat all cases of pyospermia with a combination of antibiotics and anti-inflammatory medications. It generally takes several weeks before these medications have an effect in the genital duct system and the WBC count falls.

The regimen I typically use is:

- Antibiotic for three to four weeks (sometimes as long as six weeks), either ciprofloxacin 500 mg twice a day or doxycycline 100 mg twice a day

- Anti-inflammatory medication while taking the antibiotic; I generally recommend ibuprofen 600 mg three times a day with food

Ibuprofen can be bought over the counter inexpensively; it comes in 200 mg tablets, so I tell patients to take three tablets with each meal. There is also a wide array of prescription anti-inflammatory medications that can be taken instead of ibuprofen, such as oxaprozin (Daypro) and celecoxib (Celebrex). These have the advantage of needing to be taken less often than ibuprofen. However, they are significantly more expensive and are not felt to be more effective than ibuprofen in their anti-inflammatory effect. Medications such as celecoxib are also marketed as having less gastrointestinal side effects, but they have been associated with an increased risk of cardiovascular events with prolonged use. Before taking anti-inflammatories, it is important to check with your doctor if you have a history of stomach ulcers, gastroesophageal reflux disease (GERD), or decreased kidney function or kidney disease.

It takes time for inflammation to subside, so I recommend a repeat semen analysis four to six weeks after beginning treatment for pyospermia. I'm looking for a normal WBC level, under 1 million per cc. If WBC levels are decreasing but are still above normal at the time of the retest, then a third semen analysis ten to twelve weeks later may be indicated.

Symptomatic Pyospermia

Treatment of symptomatic pyospermia is dependent on the results of the testing that was performed, such as a urinalysis or urine culture. Once the treatment is complete and the symptoms have cleared up, semen analysis is repeated six to eight weeks later. If the symptoms do not clear up, then further evaluation and treatment by a urologist is indicated.

For chlamydia or gonorrhea, the latest guidelines from the Centers for Disease Control recommend a single dose of *one* of the following:

- Ceftriaxone 250 mg by injection *or*
- Cefixime 400 mg by mouth or
- Ceftizoxime 500 mg by injection *or*
- Cefoxitin 2 g by injection along with probenecid 1 g by mouth *or*
- Cefotaxime 500 mg by injection

plus one of the following:

- Azithromycin 1 g by mouth in a single dose *or*
- Doxycycline 100 mg by mouth twice a day for seven days

If a sexually transmitted disease such as chlamydia or gonorrhea is found, the female partner should also get tested by her ob-gyn. The couple should use a condom or practice abstinence until both partners have completed their courses of treatment, to prevent spread of the infection back and forth between them.

If the urine test comes back as positive for a bacterial urinary tract infection (UTI), then the choice of antibiotic should be determined by what antibiotic the culture says the bacteria are sensitive to. Typically a ten-to-fourteen-day course of antibiotics is indicated for men, though a longer course (three to six weeks) may be necessary if the doctor suspects prostatitis as well.

Urinary tract infections are much less common in men than in women. If a man is diagnosed with a symptomatic urinary tract infection, he should see a general urologist for a basic evaluation (including a non-invasive ultrasound test to make sure that he is adequately emptying his bladder).

Persistent Pyospermia

If significant pyospermia persists following adequate treatment, then further testing is recommended to make sure that some hidden source of inflammation is not being missed, including potentially dangerous but rare problems like prostate cancer. Recommended testing includes:

- *Chlamydia and gonorrhea testing by urine test or urethral swab (if not previously done).* Diagnosis code (STD testing): V74.5 before October 2015, Z11.3 afterward. These sexually transmitted diseases can be entirely silent and without symptoms in some circumstances.

- *Transrectal ultrasound (TRUS).* Diagnosis code (prostatitis): 601.1 before October 2014, N41.9 afterward. This radiologic test provides good visualization of the prostate and seminal vesicles, and can look for abnormalities in the area such as stones or abnormal masses. Not all radiology centers offer TRUS, so you may need to call around and find one that does. Urologists also typically offer TRUS in their office.

- *Prostate-specific antigen (PSA).* Diagnosis code (PSA screening): V76.44 before October 2014, Z12.5 afterward. PSA is a screening test for prostate cancer. It is typically used in conjunction with a digital rectal exam. Prostate cancer is rare in younger men, but I have seen it in men as young as thirty. A tumor in the prostate can lead to inflammatory changes and pyospermia, depending on its location within the gland. Further evaluation by a urologist is indicated for abnormalities seen on the PSA test or ultrasound imaging. If the testing all comes back as normal, then I would recommend yearly PSA and digital rectal exam with a primary care physician or general urologist.

Semen Cultures

Some physicians advocate a semen culture in cases of persistent pyospermia, looking for aerobic and anaerobic bacteria, as well as for other organisms such as chlamydia, gonorrhea, mycoplasma, and ureaplasma. (Treatment for mycoplasma or ureaplasma is two weeks of doxycycline combined with four weeks of ciprofloxacin.) The problem with semen cultures, however, is that they are notoriously inaccurate due to the high rates of contaminated specimens. Even with thorough washing of the hands and penis with antibacterial soap prior to semen collection, the end of the urethra closest to the penile opening is still colonized by bacteria that can contaminate the specimen (but which generally do not cause fertility problems or pyospermia). In some circumstances, such as persistent pyospermia despite treatment, a semen culture might reveal antibiotic-resistant bacteria that may respond to an alternate antimicrobial regimen. However, the high rates of specimen contamination typically make interpretation of the results difficult. I recommend ordering antimicrobial sensitivity testing in these circumstances, so that any bacteria that are grown are tested for susceptibility to different antibiotics. If multiple organisms grow from the culture, then this usually represents a contaminated specimen. If a single organism grows that is resistant to the antibiotics that were used in the past, this information can help guide further treatment.

Managing Persistent Pyospermia

Persistent pyospermia sometimes cannot be eliminated completely. If the tests described above don't reveal any worrisome findings, then I put the man on antioxidants for at least three months before ordering an oxidative stress adduct (OSA) test to assess the impact of the WBCs and the oxidative stress they are causing. Reprosource offers OSA testing as part of its Advanced Semen Report (see Chapter 11 for more details).

If the OSA test results are normal, then the impact of the pyospermia on fertility should be minimal. However, if the results are abnormal, then sperm washing can be used to decrease the impact of the WBCs. WBCs have an increased impact on sperm quality the longer that they are in contact with the sperm. Therefore, immediate sperm washing after ejaculation (combined with intrauterine insemination) can minimize the time the WBCs are in contact with the sperm, possibly limiting oxidative stress damage. This is especially true if the inflammation is felt to be in the prostate region, where the sperm spend less time, though it may be less effective for epididymal inflammation, since the sperm typically spend seven to fourteen days within the epididymis during the normal maturation process.

Clumping of Sperm and Anti-Sperm Antibodies

In normal circumstances, sperm are made in what is called an "immunologically privileged" area, in which they are relatively shielded from the body's immune system. When these barriers of protection are breached, then the immune system can form antibodies against its own sperm. Some of these anti-sperm antibodies (ASAs) just float around in the bloodstream, while others can attach to the sperm itself. Usually ASAs are not clinically significant, and most men with them have no fertility problems. However, in a minority of men, these antibodies can cause problems with conceiving a child. In men who test positive for ASAs, there is currently no way to predict whether the antibodies are going to definitely cause fertility problems, other than their impact on standard semen parameters (see below).

Common causes of ASA formation include:

- Significant trauma to the scrotal region
- Genital duct infections or inflammation
- Surgery in the scrotal or genital duct region (including vasectomy)
- Genital tract obstruction
- Idiopathic (no possible causative event known)

Diagnosis of Anti-Sperm Antibodies

I suspect anti-sperm antibodies when a semen analysis shows a very low motility and/or low grade of motility along with agglutination (clumping) of sperm in which the sperm are stuck together in larger bunches. Good fertility-specific labs will comment on the presence of the sperm agglutination in a semen sample. Further testing for anti-sperm antibodies can then be done.

There are two types of testing for ASA that can be performed. In *indirect testing,* a blood test looks for the presence of circulating antibodies in the bloodstream. It's important to note that antibodies circulating in the bloodstream have *not* been found to have a significant impact on male fertility. I mention this type of testing here because it can be useful for men who have the combination of azoospermia, normal FSH, normal testicular volume, and no reason to have an obstruction (such as previous hernia repair, vasectomy, etc.). In these men, it is often unclear whether there is a sperm blockage problem or, alternatively, maturation arrest (see Chapter 9). About 70 percent of men whose azoospermia is caused by an obstruction will be positive for anti-sperm antibodies on indirect ASA testing of the blood, whereas men with nonobstructive azoospermia should not have any anti-sperm antibodies. (However, men with congenital blockages or sperm stasis problems—see Chapter 9—will likely not have elevated levels of direct ASA, as opposed to men with an acquired blockage, who usually will.) This information may help to guide treatment options, although without a testicular biopsy it cannot be definitely determined whether the problem is one of production or one of blockage.

Direct (immunobead) testing, by contrast, looks for antibodies directly attached to the sperm themselves and determines what percentage of sperm have antibodies attached to them. If 20 percent or more of the sperm have antibodies attached to them, that is generally considered significant. The type of antibody present may also be tested for, with immunoglobulin A (IgA) thought to have a more significant impact on fertility than immunoglobulin G (IgG).

Anti-Sperm Antibodies and Fertility

Anti-sperm antibodies can impact fertility in one of two ways: by decreasing sperm motility or by making it harder for the sperm to fertilize the egg.

ASAs can decrease motility by causing sperm to clump together. Clumped sperm do not swim well, and so they can have trouble traveling up the fallopian tubes to reach an egg.

The second possibility is that antibodies can attach to the head of the sperm, interfering with the normal sperm-egg interactions that are necessary for egg fertilization.

Most men (70 to 80 percent or more in some studies) who have been tested using the Indirect ASA test following a vasectomy have been found to have anti-sperm antibodies in their bloodstream. It is a common misconception that these anti-sperm antibodies significantly decrease fertility in men who have their vasectomy reversed. In reality, most men who undergo a successful vasectomy reversal have no ASA-related fertility problems afterward. There is even some evidence to suggest that vasectomy reversal may decrease or even eliminate the presence of ASAs.

Management of Anti-Sperm Antibodies

If direct (immunobead) testing shows that ASAs are impacting more than 20 percent of sperm and there is a significant decrease in sperm motility, then there are several potential treatment options.

One is to combine sperm washing with intrauterine insemination (IUI). The washing process can sometimes break up the agglutinated sperm and improve sperm motility. Before proceeding with IUI, a test wash can be done at the time of a semen analysis to see if the washing process will significantly improve motility. Small studies have shown a pregnancy rate of up to 15–30 percent when IUI is combined with sperm washing.

A second approach is via the immune system. Since antibodies against sperm are an immunologic reaction, using corticosteroids to slightly suppress the immune system should have the potential to decrease antibody levels and improve sperm quality. However, studies looking at whether this works have had mixed results. To see if there is any benefit for a particular man, a doctor can prescribe a ten-day course of prednisone (e.g. 10 mg by mouth once per day) prior to a repeat semen analysis. If significant improvements in sperm motility are seen on the new semen analysis, then the man can take prednisone 10 mg daily for days 1 through 10 of the woman's menstrual cycle (with day 1 defined as the day of first full menstrual flow). A possible alternative is for the man to take prednisone 20 mg daily for days 1 through 10 of the woman's menstrual cycle, followed by prednisone 5 mg daily for days 11 through 14 of her cycle (the lower dose serves to taper off from the higher initial dose; higher doses of corticosteroids should never be stopped abruptly).

The steroids can be used for as long as a year, with repeat semen analysis testing every three months to ensure that the man is continuing to respond to the corticosteroids. I also usually recommend that he take an anti-ulcer medication such as ranitidine (Zantac), famotidine (Pepcid), or nizatidine (Axid) while on the steroids, to decrease the risk of gastrointestinal side effects.

The use of corticosteroids is not without risks. Fortunately, severe side effects are uncommon, but it is important to be aware of them. Potential side effects include:

- Aseptic necrosis of the hip and compression fracture of bones (rare, but can necessitate hip replacement or cause permanent disability)
- Mood changes
- Altered glucose metabolism, possibly indicating diabetes
- New onset or worsening of peptic ulcer disease
- Acne
- Gastrointestinal side effects (diarrhea, bloating, increased gas)
- Weight gain
- Facial flushing
- Impaired wound healing
- Fluid retention
- High blood pressure
- Glaucoma
- Insomnia

Side effects are generally related to higher dosages and longer durations of treatment. Men with known risk factors, such as elevated blood sugar levels, glaucoma, congestive heart failure, or peptic ulcer disease, should check with their primary care physician before starting these medications.

If a test wash of the sperm does not improve sperm motility, then sometimes combining corticosteroids with sperm washing can help. A test sperm wash following a seven-to-ten-day course of prednisone 10 mg once a day can be performed to see if this results in improved sperm motility. If significant improvements are seen, then the man can take prednisone 10 mg daily for seven to ten days prior to IUI, *or* prednisone 20 mg by mouth daily for seven to ten days prior to IUI, followed by prednisone 5 mg by mouth daily for four days (to taper off the higher dosage).

If sperm washes and corticosteroids don't do the trick, then IVF/ICSI is a very effective treatment (see Appendix D). Since a single sperm is directly injected into each egg in the laboratory, the sperm do not need to swim or interact normally with the egg, and therefore the impact of any ASAs is irrelevant.

Demographic Factors That Can Impact Male Fertility

Age and being either overweight or underweight can affect a man's fertility. Read this section if you answered yes to any question in Section 2 of the Personal Fertility Profile.

Increasing Paternal Age

In recent decades, both men and women have been delaying having children until later in life. Since 1980, birth rates in the United States have increased by 40 percent for men ages thirty-five to forty-nine and decreased by 20 percent for men under thirty. For various reasons, many couples are simply choosing to wait longer to start a family than couples did in the past.

For women, there is a clear decrease in fertility as they approach the age of forty. Men do not have the same timeline for decreasing fertility potential, and stories abound of men fathering children well into their seventies and eighties. At some point, however, a man's fertility potential does begin to decrease, although the age at which this happens varies considerably; sometime between the ages of forty-five and fifty years would probably be accurate for a large percentage of men.

Causes of Aging-Associated Changes in Male Fertility

Several factors associated with aging can play a role in decreasing reproductive potential in men. These include decreased testosterone levels, increased body fat, increased oxidative stress, and chronic diseases that can affect fertility, such as diabetes, erectile dysfunction, and hypothyroidism.

Furthermore, with increasing age come elevated levels of sperm fragmentation (measured by the DNA fragmentation index, or DFI; see Chapter 11). Below you'll see how DFI changes with age; a normal DFI is under 30 percent.

Age	Average DFI
20–29	12.9%
30–39	16.3%
40–49	23.2%
50–59	35.4%
60–80	49.6%

A. J. Wyrobek et al., "Advancing Age Has Differential Effects on DNA Damage, Chromatin Integrity, Gene Mutations, and Aneuploidies in Sperm," *Proceedings of the National Academy of Sciences* 103, no. 25 (2006): 9601–6.

Changes in Semen Parameters and Natural Fertility

One clear change in semen parameters commonly seen over time is decreased ejaculate volume. As men age, their prostate and seminal vesicles make less fluid. After thirty-five years of age, sperm density, motility, and morphology generally start to decrease, but not to the point of significantly impacting fertility until about age forty-five to fifty (as opposed to women, whose relative fertility potential may have dropped by half once they reach their late thirties). Studies have shown that men forty-five and older have a four to five times greater chance of taking a year or longer to establish a pregnancy when compared to men who are twenty-five or younger. In addition, miscarriage rates tend to be higher as men age, with rates two to three times higher in men over forty-five years old as opposed to those under age thirty. Of course, there is wide individual variation due to a multitude of factors, including genetics, lifestyle choices, and general health.

Changes in IUI/IVF Outcomes

The impact of advanced paternal age on intrauterine insemination outcomes is controversial, although decreasing semen parameters in the fifth and sixth decades of a man's life would be expected to have a negative impact on pregnancy rates.

With IVF, live birth rates do seem to decrease as the father gets older, especially when the woman is older as well. Sperm DNA damage tends to be found in higher rates in older men, though a woman's eggs are known to be able to repair some degree of this damage. However, this DNA repair ability of eggs may decrease as women get older, and therefore, eggs from an older woman may be less able to repair DNA damage in sperm from older men. Supporting evidence for this comes from studies that show no difference in IVF outcomes with advancing paternal age when donor eggs from younger women are used. Other studies have shown that when ICSI is used with IVF, no significant decrease is seen in pregnancy rates in relation to paternal age when semen parameters are normal. However, in men with low sperm count (oligospermia), lower pregnancy rates for IVF/ICSI are seen as the man's age rises. Therefore, advanced paternal age seems to have a negative impact on IVF outcomes primarily when the woman is also older and when baseline semen parameters are decreased.

Increased Risk of Inherited Disorders

Traditionally, babies of older mothers are thought to have an elevated risk of birth defects. Recently, however, more attention has been focused on how the age of the father affects rates of birth defects and other developmental abnormalities. *It must be emphasized that the vast majority of older men conceive children without any genetic abnormalities or birth defects whatsoever.* What follows is a list of those disorders that are sometimes seen in the children of older fathers, albeit uncommonly.

Down Syndrome (Trisomy 21)

Older mothers have a well-described risk of having a child with Down syndrome:

Age of Mother	Risk of Down Syndrome in Child
25	1 in 1,250
35	1 in 385
40	1 in 106
45	1 in 35

With men, being older seems to have a weak but positive correlation with an increased risk of Down syndrome in offspring. The risk is compounded when the mother is older as well (over thirty).

Schizophrenia

The risk of developing schizophrenia has been shown to be higher among children of older fathers, among other factors. Men who are fifty or older have about a three times greater risk of conceiving a child who will develop schizophrenia when compared to men less than twenty-five years old (1 in 47 for older fathers compared to 1 in 147 for younger fathers).

Autism

The risk of having a child with autism appears to be correlated (at least in part) with advancing paternal age. Men age forty years and older have been found to have three or more times greater risk of having a child with autism than younger men.

Autosomal Dominant Mutations

Human beings have two copies of each chromosome, one inherited from each parent. Occasionally abnormal genes are inherited from one parent (or sometimes from both parents). Whether or not the abnormal gene will lead to a disorder in the child depends on multiple factors. Autosomal dominant disorders are chromosomal abnormalities in which only one abnormal copy of the gene is needed in order for the disease to show up. The risk of having a child with some types of these genetic abnormalities does appear to increase as the father's age rises. A forty-year-old father has about a 0.3–0.5 percent chance of conceiving children with chromosomal abnormalities, and by age fifty the risk has double that of younger men.

Examples of chromosomal disorders (autosomal dominant as well as other types) that have been shown to increase with advancing paternal age include polycystic kidney disease, achondroplasia (dwarfism), tuberous sclerosis, Alpert syndrome, Pfeiffer syndrome, and Crouzon syndrome.

Birth Defects

Being older may mildly increase the risk of fathering a child with cleft palate, diaphragmatic hernia, or right ventricular outflow tract obstruction of the heart.

Screening the Fetus for Abnormalities

Although the vast majority of older men will have normal children, there is accumulating evidence that the risk of certain abnormalities does increase with the age of the male partner. This increased risk seems to be amplified when the female partner is also older. At this point in time, there are no screening tests available to detect an elevated risk of such problems as autism or schizophrenia. Known genetic disorders can potentially be screened for using preimplantation genetic diagnosis (PGD) in conjunction with IVF (see Chapter 10). Chorionic villus sampling (at 10–12 weeks of gestation), amniocentesis (at 15–20 weeks of gestation), and percutaneous umbilical cord blood sampling (after 17 weeks of gestation) are examples of tests that can be used to look for genetic abnormalities in fetuses, in addition to routine ultrasound screening and some types of blood tests (e.g., triple screen/quad screen). With some of these tests come the disadvantages of a small increase in the risk of pregnancy loss and the difficulties associated with making decisions about whether or not to let a pregnancy progress if a significant genetic abnormality is discovered.

Weight

Obesity is a well-known risk factor for male-factor infertility. Excessive fat can have a negative effect on a man's hormone levels, increasing estradiol and decreasing FSH and LH. Levels of both free and total testosterone also are known to decrease with obesity, with the size of the decrease being proportional to the degree of obesity. Excess fat around the groin and inner thigh areas can also insulate the testicles and increase the temperature within the scrotal region; numerous research studies have shown a correlation between decreased sperm counts/sperm quality and being overweight or obese. Sexual and ejaculatory dysfunction, as well as increased levels of sperm DNA fragmentation, have also been found to be associated with carrying excessive weight.

On the other end of the spectrum, extremely thin men may have problems with sperm production as well, due to hormonal and nutritional issues. Being underweight has been associated with lower testosterone levels, increased FSH, and decreased sperm density.

From a medical standpoint, body mass index (BMI), which takes into account both height and weight, is the tool used to determine whether someone is of normal weight, overweight or obese, or underweight. You can calculate your own BMI using one of the many BMI calculators available online. An ideal BMI value is usually defined as being between 18.5 and 24.9. Because BMI measures weight in relation to height, BMI may not be accurate in heavily muscled men, so individual body characteristics do need to be taken into account. For the majority of men, however, BMI is a fairly good indicator of whether they are at a healthy weight.

Underweight (Low BMI)

As discussed previously, men with a very low BMI can have fertility problems due to abnormalities of hormones and nutritional deficiencies. Many men with a low BMI have very fast metabolisms and just cannot seem to gain weight no matter how many calories they consume. If a man has any symptoms of hyperthyroidism (sweating, palpitations, etc.) then a TSH level can be drawn to see if he has hyperthyroidism (see Chapter 4). Otherwise, the best strategy that these men can take is to eat a healthy, well-balanced diet and avoid overexercising (see Chapter 5).

Overweight or Obese (Elevated BMI)

From a fertility standpoint, gradual weight loss through a combination of increased exercise and dietary modification is generally the best way to improve fertility.

Exercise

Engaging in regular exercise—vigorous enough to moderately increase your heart rate—is a good way to help decrease weight. Men with significant health problems should check with their primary care physician before starting on an exercise regimen. See Chapter 5 for exercise recommendations.

Diet

There are dozens if not hundreds of weight loss diets out there. See Chapter 5 for dietary recommendations for men trying to conceive. Two particular weight loss diets that I find reasonable include the DASH diet and the Mediterranean diet.

The Dietary Approaches to Stop Hypertension (DASH) diet (www.dashdiet.org) was developed by the National Institutes of Health in order to help people with hypertension better control their blood pressure, but it's also a great example of a well-balanced approach to eating for anyone. The DASH diet emphasizes fruits, vegetables, whole grains, and low-fat dairy foods. It includes lean meat, fish, poultry, nuts, and beans as protein sources, and it recommends limiting sugar-sweetened foods and beverages, red meat, and added fats.

The Mediterranean diet has been shown to decrease the risk of heart disease, cancer, Parkinson's disease, and Alzheimer's disease. This eating plan emphasizes plant-based food (nuts, fruits, vegetables, whole grains, legumes), healthy fats (such as olive oil) instead of less healthy fats (such as butter), limiting red meat to no more than a few servings a month, avoiding excessive salt in favor of herbs and spices, eating fish and poultry at least twice a week, and (optionally) drinking red wine in moderation. It also emphasizes the importance of staying physically active.

Weight Loss Strategies That Can Harm Fertility

Crash diets that feature extreme calorie restriction and lead to rapid changes in body weight can result in nutritional deficiencies and increased oxidative stress on the body. These changes can have a negative impact on the pituitary's secretion of gonadotropins, decrease testosterone levels, and impair sperm production and quality.

Fad diets can also pose a problem. Dieting fads come and go—in the 1990s, for example, fats were bad and carbohydrates were good, while recently the Atkins and Paleo diets have identified carbohydrates as the enemy and labeled fats as either not unhealthful or something to be encouraged. I am certainly not going to wade into the controversies surrounding the efficacy and safety of each of these diets for the general population. However, from a fertility standpoint I do have some concerns about diets that exclude entire categories of food, such as carbohydrates. Some degree of carbohydrate intake is beneficial for normal sperm production, so extremely low-carb diets should probably be avoided by men who are trying to conceive. Men on very strict vegetarian diets can suffer from iron and zinc deficiencies, which can have a negative impact on fertility as well.

Weight loss surgery, also called bariatric surgery, can lead to substantial and sustained weight loss in many obese patients. This type of surgery has been shown to have a potentially positive impact on rates of diabetes, rates of hypertension, and life expectancy. Some studies have shown improvements in hormone profiles in obese men following bariatric surgery, but the overall impact on fertility has not been well studied. Immediately following bariatric surgery, men often have significant decreases in sperm counts (even dropping to zero) and sperm quality, despite normal hormone profiles. Potential reasons for this include problems absorbing nutrients as a result of surgical techniques that reduce the size of the stomach or bypass it, as well as the release of toxic substances as large amounts of fat are burned in a relatively short period. Over the long term, these men may well rebound and have an improved fertility status, but ongoing problems with nutrient absorption abnormalities can lead to longstanding sperm quality problems in some men.

Lifestyle-Related Fertility Issues

Sperm quality depends to a great extent on the testicular environment in which the sperm are being produced. There are a wide variety of lifestyle-related activities that can make this environment for sperm production less than ideal. Read this section if you answered yes to any question in Section 3 of the Personal Fertility Profile.

As mentioned previously, the human spermatogenic cycle is approximately ten weeks. Something that negatively affects the testicles, such as using a hot tub or sauna, can potentially have a negative effect on all of the sperm in the body at the time, and it can take ten weeks for the body to completely get rid of the old, damaged batch of sperm and get a new, undamaged batch of sperm back in the ejaculate. Along the same lines, any positive lifestyle changes that have been made (such as quitting smoking or decreasing alcohol intake) take at least one spermatogenic cycle (ten weeks, or two and a half months) and sometimes two cycles (five months) to be fully reflected in the semen parameters.

There are a number of activities that are known to decrease the quantity and/or quality of sperm. An important point to remember is that the biology of each man is different, so the impact of each of these activities can vary widely from person to person. For example, some men could sit in a sauna for four hours a day and not have any change in their semen parameters, while others could start to have significant changes after just ten minutes of sauna use. Since there is no way to determine in advance each individual's distinct response to each risk factor, I recommend avoiding all potentially detrimental activities while a couple is actively trying to conceive a pregnancy.

One final point to consider is the constant barrage of news articles in the popular media that claim to show that certain foods, supplements, or activities have been found to be associated with improvements or decreases in sperm numbers or quality. Whether it's avocados, nonstick pots and pans, or the type of laundry detergent you are using, just about everything seems to have some scientific study associated with it showing that this breakthrough finding is either your ticket to pregnancy or your ultimate barrier to conceiving. Almost all of these studies are small and uncontrolled, and have little scientific merit by themselves. In this book, I have tried to identify the risk factors and beneficial activities that have decent scientific data backing up their use or avoidance. So before you rip up your carpet (because of those nasty perfluorochemicals), throw away your bedding and sofas (because of insidious off-gassing from the flame-retardant chemicals), or stop taking showers (due to the evil phthalates in your shower curtain), read through this section to see which interventions are actually based on sound scientific findings at this time, and leave the sensationalism to the newspapers and cable TV.

Tobacco Products

Tobacco in all of its forms (cigarettes, cigars, chewing tobacco, snuff) can be detrimental to fertility, not to mention a man's general health. Although nicotine by itself is thought to have a mild negative impact on fertility, by far the greatest impact is from other toxic chemicals in tobacco, including polycyclic aromatic hydrocarbons, vinyl chloride, and benzoprene, to name a few. These dangerous substances are known to negatively affect fertility in several ways, including having a direct toxic effect on sperm production, increasing oxidative stress on the body, and creating hormonal disturbances that can disrupt the normal balance between the pituitary gland and the testicles. Numerous studies have linked tobacco to decreases in sperm production and sperm quality. IVF success rates have also been shown to be reduced in smokers as well.

Because nicotine is highly addictive, it's typically very difficult to quit smoking. You can get help with stopping smoking from medications that help decrease cravings for nicotine, such as bupropion (Zyban) or varenicline (Chantix); through programs such as the American Lung Association's Freedom from Smoking program (www.ffsonline.org); by working with a psychotherapist; or by using nicotine replacement products, which are available over the counter.

Nicotine replacement therapy can help to satisfy the cravings for nicotine while avoiding the toxic byproducts of tobacco. It is often used in addition to one or more of the other smoking cessation techniques listed above. In some cases people slowly wean themselves off the nicotine replacement; other people simply use the nicotine replacements long-term, but avoiding tobacco products. As mentioned above, nicotine by itself has been found in some studies to potentially have a mild negative effect on male fertility, but eliminating the other chemicals—more than two thousand of them—found in tobacco can only benefit a man's fertility potential. If nicotine replacement is needed to achieve this, then it is well worth the trade-off in terms of the small potential negative impact of nicotine itself.

Nicotine replacement comes in various formats, including gum, inhalers, lozenges, patches, nasal spray, and electronic cigarettes. Electronic cigarettes have proven to be quite effective with my patients, as they both satisfy the nicotine cravings and provide the familiar feeling of having a cigarette in the mouth. Many e-cigarettes also have ways to gradually taper the amount of nicotine that is delivered, which can help to achieve eventual cessation.

Illicit Drugs

Essentially all illegal drugs, such as marijuana, heroin, cocaine, and so on, have been shown to have a negative impact on male fertility. These negative effects include decreased testosterone levels, lower sperm production and quality, negative effects on the interaction between sperm and egg, erectile dysfunction, and ejaculatory problems. For these reasons, I recommend that men wishing to establish a pregnancy stop the use of all illegal drugs.

Alcohol

Moderate alcohol intake in men has not been found to have a significant negative impact on fertility when studied across large populations. However, greater amounts of alcohol intake can both have a direct toxic effect on sperm production and produce hormonal abnormalities (such as lower testosterone, elevated FSH, and elevated estradiol) that negatively affect sperm numbers and quality. The more alcohol a man drinks, the greater the potential negative effect. The general recommendation for men who are trying to have children is to limit their alcohol intake to no more than four drinks per week.

Activities That Generate Excessive Heat

The testicles are located outside of the body because they like to be two to three degrees cooler than the rest of the body for optimal sperm production. The body has many effective mechanisms to keep scrotal temperature at ideal levels, and it can handle most weather- and exercise-related heat changes. In general, for every one-degree increase in ambient temperature, the scrotal temperature increases by only about a tenth as much. Still, despite these effective mechanisms, the testicles can be exposed to amounts of heat that cause problems with fertility. In fact, certain professions in which workers are routinely exposed to higher temperatures—bakers, chefs, ceramic oven operators, glassblowers, welders, and so on—are associated with higher levels of heat-related male fertility issues.

How hot is too hot? There is no set answer to this that applies to everybody. As with any other male-factor issue, it varies by individual. However, studies have shown that taking a fairly hot bath or shower—over 104°F—can cause a reduction in sperm count or sperm quality in some men. For comparison, 104°F is often pre-set as the water temperature for many hot tubs. Temperatures in saunas are often above 150°F.

I recommend that men trying to have children avoid hot tubs, saunas, and hot baths, and to take warm but not hot showers.

There are other potentially problematic causes of heat exposure that you may not have thought of. For example, lots of people use laptop computers directly on their lap. But some studies have shown that in as little as 10 minutes this can create enough heat to decrease semen parameters in some men. If you use a laptop, put it on a desk or put a thick barrier (such as a pillow) between the laptop and your lap, so that you don't feel any excess heat. Car seat warmers are another potential source of heat exposure. Don't use them if you're trying to conceive. And remember that the life cycle of sperm is about ten weeks, so if you've been exposed to any of these sources of heat, sperm quality may be impacted for the next two and a half months.

Boxers or Briefs?

This topic can be controversial, with different research articles showing findings that support both sides of the argument. Wearing tight underpants does appear to inhibit one of the body's most effective natural mechanisms for scrotal temperature control. Normally, when the scrotum gets hot it stretches out, which increases its surface area. This both decreases scrotal temperature directly and provides a greater surface area for sweat to evaporate from, which also has a cooling effect. Tight underpants keep the scrotum from effectively expanding, and also press it against the warm body and inner thighs.

Wearing tight underpants shouldn't make much of a difference for men who live and work in cool, temperature-controlled environments. However, for men who spend a fair amount of time in warmer temperatures, tighter underpants can pose a problem, and for them I suggest boxers. Also, boxers may be of benefit to men in jobs that have significant heat exposure.

What about boxer briefs, which are not necessarily tight but do provide some support in the scrotal area? It depends on how the boxer briefs fit that particular man and the fabric out of which they are made. If the boxer-briefs are fairly tight and do not allow the scrotum to descend much when exposed to heat, then switching to regular boxers may be a good idea if you have significant heat exposure during the day.

Cell Phone Use

Cell phones generate electromagnetic radiation, and some scientific studies have showed a negative impact on semen parameters with cell phone use of over four hours per day. However, it remains unclear whether regular cell phone use (where the cell phone is held up to the ear) can significantly impact sperm quality, since the radiation generated by these devices generally travels only a short distance.

I feel that the bigger concern is when cell phones are carried near the scrotum. When cell phone radiation is near the scrotum, it has been shown to increase oxidative stress in the region of the testicles as well as affect the functioning of the mitochondria (cellular energy generators) in nearby cells. The Environmental Working Group reviewed ten research studies on the topic and found that significant changes in sperm density and motility were associated with men who kept their cellular phones in the their pants pockets or on their belts. This group came up with four recommendations to decrease cell-phone-related radiation exposure to the scrotum:

- Text more, talk less. Phones emit less radiation with texting than calling.
- Don't bother with radiation shields. These shields—antenna caps or keypad covers—reduce the connection quality and force the phone to use more energy (and emit more radiation).
- If using a headset, hold the phone away from your body, not in your pants pocket or clipped to your belt. As the phone seeks to keep a constant connection between it and the headset, it creates a zone of radiation around the scrotal area.
- Call when the signal is strong. Radiation exposure increases significantly when the cell phone signal is weak.

The key issue with cell phones is how close they are to the scrotum while in use. The amount of radiation absorbed by the body decreases dramatically with even small increases in the distance of the cell phone from the body. It's fine to keep a cell phone that is completely turned off in your front pants pocket. However, if the phone is on, then the farther away it is from the scrotum, the better. You'll get the most radiation exposure if the phone is on and in your front pants pocket (and it's even worse to be talking on a Bluetooth headset at the same time). Second worst is having the cell phone clipped to a belt or in the back pocket. Slightly better would be storing it in a lower pants pocket (like in cargo pants). The best idea is to keep the cell phone in a coat pocket, shirt pocket, bag, or briefcase while carrying it around.

Lubricant Use During Intercourse

Trying to conceive a child can be stressful for couples, and this stress can contribute to vaginal dryness in some women. Many couples assume that lubricants that do not contain spermicidal agents are okay to use when trying to conceive, but unfortunately most vaginal lubricants are detrimental to sperm quality when they come into contact with sperm. Lubricants can impact sperm in multiple ways, including decreasing their motility, elevating levels of DNA fragmentation, and decreasing their ability to survive.

Lubricants that have little to minimal impact on sperm quality and function include:

- Pre-Seed (this seems to be the best according to current studies)
- Conceive Plus
- Baby oil or canola oil

Lubricants that may have a negative impact on sperm quality and function include:

- Astroglide
- KY lubricants (including Sensitive, Warming, and Tingling)
- Saliva

- Surgical gels (such as Surgilube)
- Olive oil or sesame oil
- Replens
- Lubrins
- Maybe Baby
- Yes
- Forelife
- Sylk
- Petroleum jelly (such as Vaseline)
- Femglide
- Lubifax
- Keri lotion

I don't think there's good evidence that some lubricants can actually increase the chances of conception. However, couples who require lubrication for comfortable intercourse should choose Pre-Seed, Conceive Plus, baby oil, or canola oil.

Caffeine

Most studies have shown that caffeine intake does not have a negative impact on semen parameters. However, some studies have suggested a possible negative effect if daily caffeine intake exceeds 800 mg. Take a look at the average amounts of caffeine in common beverages:

Drink	Average caffeine content
Percolated coffee	100 mg per 6 oz. cup
Drip coffee	145 mg per 6 oz. cup
Espresso	100 mg per 1 oz. shot
Black tea	50 mg per 8 oz cup
Cola	35 mg per 12 oz. can
Mountain Dew	54 mg per 12 oz. can
Red Bull	80 mg per 8.5 oz. can

As long as caffeine intake does not exceed 800 mg per day, it probably will not have a significant negative impact on fertility.

Exercise

Moderate exercise is recommended for optimizing a man's fertility potential, but excessive bicycle riding has been associated with decreases in sperm counts and quality. See "Exercise" in Chapter 5 for more information.

Soy

Soy contains phytoestrogens, substances that are known to have estrogenic effects. Though controversial, some studies have suggested a decrease in sperm counts and quality in men who regularly eat soy products. See "Is Soy a Problem?" in Chapter 5.

Job-Related Factors

Section 4 of the Personal Fertility Profile reviews job-related factors that can impact the fertility potential of some men. Read this section if you answered yes to any of those questions.

Sitting for Prolonged Periods of Time

Many jobs in today's modern economy involve sitting for long periods of time, whether in front of a computer terminal at a desk or in the cab of a long-distance truck. Prolonged sitting can increase the scrotal temperature to the point where sperm quality can become compromised in some men. When you're sitting, the legs generally aren't free to spread much; this traps the scrotum between the thighs, which can increase the scrotal temperature significantly. The position of the scrotum between the thighs can also prevent the normal relaxation of the scrotal skin, which the body uses to regulate scrotal temperature.

Studies have shown that the scrotal temperature can increase as much as 3 to 4°F when men drive for more than two hours at a time. Higher levels of semen abnormalities have been found in men who drive for long periods, such as taxi drivers. Longer times to pregnancy have also been shown to be associated with driving more than three hours per day.

If you sit for long periods of time, whether at a desk or while driving, wear loose-fitting underpants (such as boxers) and try to sit with your legs apart to increase air flow to the scrotal area. It may also be beneficial to get up and walk around for a few minutes every hour and a half to two hours during the day. While some men attempt to decrease scrotal temperature further with ice packs in the scrotal area (there's a product out there called Snowballs— www.snowballsunderwear.com) or fanning air on the scrotal region, there's no solid evidence at this time that these approaches significantly improve male fertility.

Heat Exposure at Work

In addition to the heat-related problems that are described for men who sit for prolonged periods of time at work, men who work in other professions have significant heat exposure as well. Examples include chefs, bakers, ceramic oven operators, glassblowers, welders, and the crew of submarines, to name a few. The best intervention is letting the body's natural cooling mechanisms work as efficiently as possible by wearing boxers or other loose under-pants that allow the scrotum to stretch and increase the surface area for the evaporation of sweat.

Elevated Levels of Stress

Trying to have a child can be a stressful and emotional time. Stress can certainly have a negative effect on sexual function, causing a drop in libido and problems with getting and maintaining an erection. Studies have also shown that stress can impact fertility in some men as well (though typically to a lesser degree than the impact on women's fertility). Stress has been shown to decrease the responsiveness of the pituitary gland to gonadotropin-releasing hormone (GnRH) in some men. This can lead to decreases in LH and FSH, hormones needed for normal testicular function, with corresponding drops in testosterone and sperm production. Elevated levels of another stress-related hormone, cortisol, may also impair fertility potential.

A 2010 study by A. L. Gollenberg and colleagues, published in *Fertility and Sterility*, of 950 men trying to have a child showed that a man who experienced two or more stressful events (such as job loss, serious illness, serious legal trouble, financial strains, relationship problems, etc.) had a 1.54 to 2 times increased risk of having abnormal sperm counts, motility, or morphology. Furthermore, the men were just as affected by stressful events that happened to their female partners as they were if they themselves experienced the stressful event.

Strategies for dealing with stress include getting enough exercise, eating a healthful diet and making other healthful lifestyle choices, relaxation techniques (such as meditation), and counseling (individual or couples).

For more information about stress management, a good Internet source is WebMD (www.webmd.com).

Occupational Exposure to Toxic Chemicals

According to the National Institute for Occupational Safety and Health (NIOSH), more than a thousand chemicals used in the workplace have been associated with reproductive side effects in animals, although human studies are lacking for most of these substances. An additional four million other commercially used chemicals have not been studied at all.

Some chemicals that have known or suspected negative impacts on male fertility include:

- *Heavy metals and other elements.* Jobs with significant exposure to elements such as lead, cadmium, boron, and mercury include welding; factory work making chemicals or using heavy metals; making jewelry, ceramics, or stained glass; and painting (using lead-based paint).

- *Polychlorinated biphenyls.* PCBs are often found in capacitors, electric motors, and transformers.

- *Industrial solvents.* Solvents (such as carbon disulfide, among many others) are commonly used in industry, but they can lead to hormonal changes and decreases in semen quality in some men. They are frequently found in paints, varnishes, lacquers, adhesives, glues, degreasers, cleaning and agents, and they are often used in the production of dyes, polymers, plastics, textiles, printing inks, agricultural products, pharmaceuticals.

- *Pesticides, herbicides, and fungicides.* Agricultural and greenhouse workers, who are often exposed to these chemicals, have been found to have decreased semen parameters.

- *Plastic components.* Chemicals such as phthalates and bisphenols, often used in plastics, are known to be endocrine disruptors or weak estrogens.

NIOSH lists the following recommendations for limiting potential toxic exposure to workplace chemicals:

1. Store chemicals in sealed containers when not in use.
2. Wash hands before eating, drinking, or smoking.
3. Avoid skin contact with chemicals.

4. If chemicals do come into contact with the skin, follow the directions for washing provided in the material safety data sheet (MSDS) for the chemical, which should be available through your workplace.

5. Become familiar with the chemicals used in your workplace that pose potential reproductive hazards.

6. To prevent workplace chemicals from contaminating the home:

   - Change out of contaminated clothing and wash with soap and water before going home.

   - Store street clothes in a separate area of the workplace to prevent contamination.

   - Wash work clothing separately from other laundry (at work, if possible).

   - Avoid bringing home clothing or other objects that may be contaminated.

   - Participate in all safety and health education, training, and monitoring programs offered by your employer.

   - Learn about proper work practices, engineering controls, and personal protective equipment (i.e., gloves, respirators, and personal protective clothing) that can be used to reduce exposures to hazardous substances.

   - Follow the safety and health work practices and procedures implemented by your employer.

Air Pollution

Air pollution can come from many different sources, including car exhaust, industrial production, and the burning of coal and wood. There are thousands of potential toxins involved with air pollution, with some of the more common ones being carbon monoxide, sulfur dioxide, and ozone. Significant exposure to air pollution has been linked to decreases in sperm quality as well as increased sperm DNA damage.

Strategies for reducing exposure to air pollution include limiting outdoor activity when local air quality conditions are poor and trying to avoid traffic-congested streets if possible. When driving in traffic, keep the windows up and use the "recirculate" setting on your car, to avoid bringing in more outside air than necessary.

Medications and Supplements

As we've seen, sperm production is a complex process that lasts approximately ten weeks, during which time sperm precursor cells are transformed into fully mature sperm. At any time during this process, sperm production can be influenced by outside factors, including medications or supplements you may be taking.

Section 5 of the Personal Fertility Profile reviews the impact of certain prescription medications and nonprescription supplements on male fertility. If you answered yes to any of the questions in that section of the profile, review this section to see if they may be impacting your fertility potential.

Prescription Medications

The following categories of medications are known to potentially have a significant negative impact on male fertility:

- Antibiotics
- Antifungal/antiparasitic medications
- Antiseizure medications
- Cardiovascular medications
- Chemotherapeutic agents
- Gastrointestinal medications
- Gout medications
- Hormonally active agents

- Narcotics/opiates
- Prostate medications
- Psychiatric medications

I'll discuss each of these, and at the end I'll mention some other medications that don't fall into any of the preceding categories. You should be aware that this is not a complete list, either; studies are constantly being performed to identify additional medications that can affect fertility.

It is important that you have a discussion with your health care provider before making any changes to your medications. This book aims to provide you with information for your own knowledge, and you can share it with your personal physician if you learn something that may be pertinent to your situation. Decisions about which medications are right for you depend heavily upon individual factors, and the potential risks or benefits to stopping or changing any of your medications need to be adequately weighed by a health care professional familiar with your medical history and circumstances.

Antibiotics

Many antibiotics are known to have a potentially negative impact on sperm quality. These include:

- Tetracycline
- Aminoglycosides (such as erythromycin, gentamicin, and neomycin)
- Nitrofurantoin
- Minocycline
- Sulfamethoxazole (Septra, Bactrim), co-trimoxazole
- Penicillin
- Ampicillin

Antifungals and Antiparasitics

Some antifungal and antiparasitic medications are known to have a potentially negative impact on sperm quality. These include:

- Ketoconazole
- Chloroquine
- Niridazole

Antiseizure Medications

Although antiseizure medications such as carbamazepine (Tegretol) are known to be associated with decreased testosterone levels and sperm quality in some men, these medications cannot typically be safely stopped due to the health and safety risks involved with recurrent uncontrolled seizures. Epilepsy itself may also be related to hormonal imbalances in some men.

Cardiovascular Medications

There are many types of medications that are used to treat various cardiovascular problems, and some of them may have an effect on fertility in men:

- Spironolactone: can decrease testosterone levels and negatively impact sperm function
- Calcium channel blockers: may interfere with egg/sperm interactions
- Digoxin: may affect erections and libido
- Clonidine: can increase the chance of erectile dysfunction
- Beta-blockers: can increase the chance of erectile dysfunction
- Thiazide diuretics: can increase the chance of erectile dysfunction

Initial human studies of atorvastatin (Lipitor) showed decreased sperm motility, but no significant impact was seen in larger studies, so it is likely okay to use it to control high cholesterol.

Chemotherapeutic Agents

See "Cancer Treatment" later in this chapter for information about the impact of chemotherapy on male fertility.

Gastrointestinal Medications

A number of drugs used to treat gastrointestinal problems may be problematic for men trying to conceive. I've listed some potential alternatives.

- Cimetidine (Tagamet)
  Potential alternatives: ranitidine (Zantac), famotidine (Pep-cid), omeprazole (Prilosec)
- Metoclopramide (Reglan)
  Potential alternative: prochlorperazine (Compazine)
- Sulfasalazine (Azulfidine)
  Potential alternative: mesalamine (Asacol)

One medication that differing opinions exist about is azathioprim (Imuran), which is used for treatment of Crohn's disease (and also for treatment of rheumatoid arthritis). It may cause a small decrease in sperm motility and a mild increase in sperm DNA fragmentation. It also may have a possible mild mutagenic effect, but animal studies suggest that this is more likely to cause a slight increase in early embryonic death, as opposed to increased birth defects in children who are born.

Gout Medications

Colchicine and allopurinol, two medications used to treat gout, may have an impact on male fertility. Potential alternatives for treating this condition include probenecid, NSAIDs, corticosteroids, and dietary modification.

Hormonally Active Agents

Medications that impact hormone levels can have a significant negative impact on sperm production and quality. Examples of these medications include:

- *Exogenous androgens.* See the section on these later in this chapter.

- *Treatments for advanced prostate cancer.* Drugs such as cyproterone, leuprolide (Lupron), goserelin (Zoladex), and bicalutamide (Casodex) can decrease testosterone production.

- *Estrogen therapy.* This may decrease sperm function and potentially increase the risk of testicular cancer.

Narcotics/Opiates

Long-term narcotic use is known to have a significant negative impact on testosterone levels in most men, which can in turn have a negative impact sperm production and quality. Examples of commonly used pharmaceutical narcotics include:

- Codeine (Tylenol #3, Paramol, Nurofen Plus)
- Hydrocodone (Vicodin, Norco, Lorcet, Lortab)
- Oxycodone (OxyContin, Percocet, Roxicodone, Tylox)
- Morphine (Duramorph, Avinza, Kadian)
- Fentanyl (Durogesic, Actiq)
- Methadone

Prostate Medications

Possible negative effects may be found with the following:

- Alpha-blockers such as tamsulosin (Flomax), silodosin (Rapaflo): may cause anejaculation or retrograde ejaculation (see those sections later in this chapter)

- 5-alpha reductase inhibitors such as finasteride (Proscar), dutasteride (Avodart): some studies have found a mild increase in the risk of ejaculatory and erectile dysfunction with these medications, as well as the potential for hormonal imbalances

- Saw palmetto (herbal supplement): may act like 5-alpha reductase inhibitors (above) and cause similar problems

Psychiatric Medications

Some antidepressant medications, especially the selective serotonin reuptake inhibitors (SSRIs), such as fluoxetine (Prozac), paroxetine (Paxil), sertraline (Zoloft), citalopram (Celexa), and escitalopram (Lexapro), can be problematic for men trying to conceive. They may be associated with erectile dysfunction and ejaculatory dysfunction (see the sections on these later in this chapter). They may cause a longer sperm transit time, which can lead to decreased sperm motility, increased sperm DNA fragmentation, and in rare cases azoospermia (which studies show resolved one month after stopping the medication).

Some studies have shown fewer sperm transport issues with a change in antidepressants from SSRIs to medications such as bupropion (Wellbutrin). Of course, the mental well-being of the man needs to be taken into consideration as well, and any changes to antidepressant medications should only be made under the careful monitoring of a primary care physician or psychiatrist.

Antipsychotic medications such as haloperidol, benperidol, and trifluperidol can modestly decrease sperm production and quality in some men. These medications can be difficult and/or unsafe to modify, and changes should be made only under the care of a primary care physician or psychiatrist.

Other Medications That Can Affect Sperm Production

A number of other drugs may cause fertility-related problems in men:

- Cyclosporine: used to prevent rejection in organ transplantation, it can decrease sperm quality in some men.

- Danazol: a weak androgen sometimes used to treat angi-oedema. Its effects on fertility are not clear at this time.

- Isotretinoin (Accutane): an acne drug that can decrease sperm production. Note that while women taking it are at serious risk of having a child with birth defects should they become pregnant while on the drug, men taking it do not run the same risks of birth defects in children they may father while on it.

- Methotrexate: a chemotherapeutic agent used for leukemia, rheumatoid arthritis, and psoriasis. It may have a potential negative impact on sperm quality as well as a potential increase in birth defects. See "Cancer Treatment" later in this chapter.

- PDE-5 inhibitors: used for the treatment of erectile dysfunction. See "Erectile Dysfunction" later in this chapter.

- Finasteride (Propecia): used in the treatment of male pattern hair loss. This drug can potentially have a negative impact on erections, ejaculation, and the hormonal environment for sperm production. An alternative that could be used is minoxidil (Rogaine).

- Rapamycin and sirolimus: used in treatment of certain cancers and some benign vascular disorders. There is some evidence that these drugs can potentially decrease sperm counts and testosterone levels.

Herbal Medications and Supplements

Herbal medications are widely used in the United States; many people believe that these "natural" remedies have a lower risk of adverse side effects. Many men with fertility problems turn to herbal medications. A 2004 study looked at 481 men evaluated in an infertility clinic and found that 31 percent of them were taking alternative medications, and that 17 percent of these supplements had clear hormonal activity that was potentially detrimental to sperm production.

I recommend that men with fertility problems stop taking natural supplements. This is not to say that I believe there are no supplements that may eventually be found to have a beneficial impact on sperm counts and quality. Rather, at this time there are multiple problems with the way that natural supplements are tested, manufactured, and marketed.

You may think what you want about vast federal bureaucracies and their inevitable political squabblings and inefficiencies, but the FDA does provide a very powerful and beneficial service in terms of securing a degree of safety and fraud prevention with the manufacture, marketing, and distribution of prescription medications. The days of snake-oil salesmen peddling ineffective and sometimes dangerous homemade remedies are thankfully behind us, at least when it comes to medications requiring a prescription.

Unfortunately, natural supplements do not fall under the jurisdiction of the FDA, and therefore they do not undergo the same intense level of scrutiny that prescription medications need to pass before being approved for use. The criteria for safety and efficacy testing are much less stringent with natural supplements. When it comes to male fertility, a huge number of alternative treatments, ranging from specific natural supplements to eating more avocados or oysters, have been found by small, uncontrolled studies to potentially be associated with an improvement in semen parameters. In the field of prescription medications, most medications that small, uncontrolled studies have suggested may have some positive effects are later, after being tested in the much larger, more rigorous studies required to attain FDA approval, shown not to have a significant positive outcome. Natural supplements, however, do not have to undergo these larger studies, and therefore claims from these small studies are rarely proven or disproven. These small studies also do not produce the same kind of safety data seen with larger, more rigorous studies.

The other problem with a lack of FDA oversight is that the manufacturing process is much less stringently regulated for nonprescription substances. Therefore, purity and amounts of active ingredient can vary significantly between products from different manufacturers. Another alarming trend is the undisclosed addition of certain pharmaceutical agents into allegedly "natural" supplements. Sildenafil (Viagra) has been found in supposedly natural nonprescription supplements for erectile dysfunction, for example, and testosterone derivatives have been found in supposedly natural bodybuilding supplements.

In addition, many natural substances (such as root and bark extracts) have not been thoroughly studied, and may in fact contain hormonally active chemicals that are actually detrimental to male fertility.

Even if you're taking supplements for other reasons besides fertility, I strongly recommend that you stop taking them when you are trying to have a child. Some studies have shown that commonly used herbal supplements such as St. John's wort, echinacea, and ginkgo biloba may have a negative impact on male fertility.

The argument can be made that large scientific studies are expensive, and no company is going to spend the money to conduct these studies on natural supplements for which a patent cannot be obtained. I think that there may be a role for government financial support of such studies for particularly promising supplements. However, until larger controlled studies show measurable and reproducible improvements in fertility, I do not feel that these supplements are worth the money or the risk of potentially negative side effects.

Exogenous Androgens

Hypogonadism (low testosterone, or "low T") is a common problem that is being increasingly diagnosed by the medical community, primarily due to an increased awareness of the problem. Some studies have shown that as many as 20 percent of men being treated for fertility issues have hormone problems such as low testosterone. Normalization of testosterone levels can potentially result in improvements in energy, libido, sexual function, and fertility. However, the types of hormonal treatment that a man chooses to use can have a dramatic impact on his fertility.

When a man has low testosterone levels, there are two ways in which they can be increased: exogenous androgen replacement, in which testosterone is given through pills, patches, gels, injections, or pellets, and endogenous testosterone production, which involves giving a medication that causes the man's own testicles to increase their production of testosterone.

Both of these approaches effectively increase blood testosterone levels. However, sperm production is dependent upon high testosterone levels within the testicles, not just in the bloodstream. Therefore, if a man is trying to have a child, medications that increase endogenous testosterone production should be used.

Exogenous androgens, on the other hand, cause the pituitary gland to decrease the release of FSH and LH. Without sufficient FSH and LH, testicular production of testosterone and sperm dramatically decreases, with significant negative implications for male fertility. See "Testosterone" in Chapter 4 for more information.

Exogenous androgens come in four basic types: prescription testosterone replacement therapy, anabolic steroids, prohormones, and T boosters.

Prescription Testosterone Replacement

Over the last decade, there has been a significant increase in awareness and treatment of low T in men. Many people are now aware that certain aging-related problems in men, such as decreased libido, erectile dysfunction, decreased lean body mass, and osteoporosis, are associated with decreased testosterone levels and are at least partially reversible with testosterone replacement therapy. Between 2008 and 2013, there was a 170 percent increase in testosterone prescriptions written in the United States. Most of these prescriptions are for older men in whom fertility is not a concern. However, as part of this trend of increasing usage, more young men are being prescribed exogenous T replacement as well, typically without the doctor knowing of its significant negative impact on male fertility. Most men who receive exogenous T replacement wind up with sperm counts of under 1 million sperm per cc after just three to four months of therapy.

Types of Exogenous Prescription Therapy

Injections		
Testosterone cypionate (Depo-Testosterone)	Average dose: 200 mg every other week	
Testosterone enanthate (Delatestryl)	Average dose: 200 mg every other week	
Testosterone undecanoate (Aveed)	Average dose: 750 mg to start, repeated 4 weeks later, then every 10 weeks thereafter	Approved by FDA in 2014.
Transdermal gel		
Androgel 1.62%	Average dose: 40.5 mg/day (range: 20.25–81 mg/day)	
Androgel 1%	Average dose: 5 g/day (range: 2.5–10 g/day)	
Fortesta 2%	Average dose: 40 mg/day (range: 10–70 mg/day)	
Testim 1%	Average dose: 5 g/day (range: 5–10 g/day)	Some evidence shows Testim is absorbed better than Androgel, but it has an odor some men do not like.
Vogelxo	Available in 5 gm tubes/packets and pump delivering 12.5 mg per actuation	Approved by FDA in 2014.
Patch		
Androderm	Average dose: 4 mg/day (range: 2–6 mg/day)	
Testoderm TTS	Average dose: 5 mg/day	
Testoderm	Average dose: 4–5 mg/day	
Topical solution		
Axiron	Average dose: 60 mg (range: 30–120 mg/day)	
Buccal patch		
Striant	Average dose: 30 mg twice a day	
Subcutaneous pellet		
Testopel	Average dose: 150-450 mg every 3–6 months	
Nasal gel		
Natesto	11 mg three times a day	Approved by FDA in 2014.
Oral Testosterone		
Andriol	Average dose: 120–160 mg/day for the first 2–3 weeks, then 40–120 mg/day	Not supposed to have the liver toxicity associated with other oral testosterones. Currently not available in US; is available in Canada.

Side effects of prescription testosterone include:

- Acne

- Gynecomastia (breast enlargement)

- Fluid retention

- Sleep apnea (though not all experts agree on this)

- Testicular atrophy

- Erythrocytosis (increase in red blood cells as a percentage of total blood volume; can make the blood more viscous and lead to heart attack or stroke)

Anabolic Steroids

Anabolic steroids are androgens that are particularly effective at increasing muscle and bone mass. They accomplish this by promoting protein metabolism and storage.

There are some legitimate medical uses for anabolic steroids, including the treatment of anemia and to reverse protein loss in patients who have prolonged immobilization following severe illness, trauma, or surgery. Anabolic steroids are also used for appetite stimulation and maintenance of muscle mass in patients with diseases such as cancer and AIDS.

Most commonly, however, anabolic steroids are used illicitly by bodybuilders and athletes to increase muscle mass and strength, and also by athletes to help speed their recovery following sports-related injuries. Some take oral forms, such as oxymetholone (Anadrol), oxandrolone (Anavar, Oxandrin), stanozolol (Winstrol), or methandrostenolone (Dianabol, also called "Dbol"). Others use injections of nadrolone decanoate (Deca-Durabolin, also called "Deca"), nandrolone phenpropionate (Durabolin), or Boldenone undecylenate (Equipoise). There's also an ointment form, tetrahydrogestrinone (known as THG, "the cream," or "the clear").

All anabolic steroids, however, still have androgenic hormonal activity as well. Men who abuse anabolic steroids for bodybuilding purposes often take the equivalent of as much as 5,000 mg of testosterone per week, an amount far greater than the body naturally produces. The result is blood testosterone levels than can be up to twenty times higher than what is considered normal. As discussed above, high blood levels of testosterone cause the pituitary gland to decrease the release of FSH and LH, which causes testicular production of testosterone and sperm to drop significantly.

The use of anabolic steroids is banned by all major sports leagues because of the unfair competitive advantage these substances provide. Anabolic steroids are listed as controlled substances, which means that it is technically illegal to possess these substances without a prescription. Production and distribution by non-physicians is also illegal, and therefore most anabolic steroids used for non-medical reasons are manufactured in other countries and smuggled into the United States. This makes quality control and safe manufacturing supervision by such agencies as the FDA not possible.

Anabolic steroid users commonly believe that warnings about the risk of anabolic steroid use are overblown and exaggerated. However, the use of anabolic steroids is associated with many potential side effects, including:

- High blood pressure
- Erythrocytosis (increase in red blood cells as a percentage of total blood volume; can make the blood more viscous and lead to heart attack or stroke)
- Gynecomastia (breast enlargement)
- Abnormal cholesterol levels
- Blood sugar control problems

- Acne
- Increased male-pattern baldness
- Increased risk of low testosterone levels later in life

Anabolic steroids have also been linked to an increased risk of coronary artery disease as well as potential direct damage to left ventricular heart function. Liver damage and failure are other serious conditions seen with oral anabolic steroid use. Mood disorders have also been found to be more common in users of anabolic steroids.

It's estimated that more than a million men in the United States have used anabolic steroids for non-medical reasons at some point. True rates of usage are difficult to determine, as studies have shown that over half of men who use anabolic steroids for non-medical reasons do not tell their physicians they're using these substances. However, the impact of anabolic steroid use on male fertility is quite clear, with almost all men suffering a significant negative impact on sperm production and quality. It is therefore very important for all men using anabolic steroids to report their use to their fertility doctor if they are trying to conceive.

Prohormones

Prohormones are precursors to androgens. Prohormones have minimal hormone activity themselves, but they are converted by the body's metabolic processes into active androgens. Interest in prohormones increased following the Anabolic Steroid Control Act of 1990, which made anabolic steroids controlled substances in the United States. Through the use of prohormones such as andros-tenedione, 4-androstenediol, 1-androstenediol, and 19-norandrostenedione, bodybuilders and athletes found a way to use androgenic compounds legally. In an attempt to close this loophole, the Anabolic Steroid Act of 2004 included prohormones on the list of illegal anabolic steroids.

Since 2004, producers of prohormones have taken several different strategies to keep their products on the market. One (illegal) strategy is to use estrogen derivatives (which are not particularly effective at increasing muscle mass) and illicitly add other undeclared anabolic steroids to these. A second approach is the use of plant-based phytoandrogens (plant substances with androgenic actions), which are currently available over the counter in the United States. Examples of phytoandrogens include triterpenoids and pine pollen. A third approach is through the use of "designer steroids" that are specifically produced to bypass the legal restrictions on anabolic steroids and prohormones, while maintaining androgenic and anabolic actions. Some examples of these designer steroids include Helladrol or H-Drol (4-chloro-17a-methyl-androsta-1,4-diene-3,17-diol), Methastadrol or M-Drol (2a, 17a-dimethyl-etiocholan-3-one, 17b-ol), Epi-MAX (2a, 3a-epithio-17a-methyl-17b-hydroxy-5a-androstane), and 11-OXO (adrenosterone).

Controversy continues to surround prohormones in regards to their legality and effectiveness. From a fertility perspective, however, little controversy exists. The goal of prohormones is to mimic the effects of other exogenous androgens, which have a known significantly negative impact on male fertility.

DHEA

Dehydroepiandrosterone, or DHEA, is a hormone precursor to testosterone that is naturally produced by the body. It was exempted from the Anabolic Steroid Control Act of 2004 due to its designation as an "old dietary ingredient." It is therefore legally for sale in the United States as a dietary supplement, but its use is banned in organized sports competitions. DHEA has some degree of direct exogenous androgenic activity, and therefore should be avoided in men trying to conceive a child.

T Boosters

T boosters are substances that are supposed to increase the natural production of testosterone by the body. The most common use of T boosters is in men using anabolic steroids who want to promote the return of natural testosterone production between anabolic cycles. Commonly used T boosters include *Tribulus terrestris* (also known as puncture vine), ginseng (from the *Panax* genus), and D-aspartic acid (DAA), an amino acid. Examples of commercially available T boosters include Perform, T-Force, Testogen XR, and Testopro, among many others.

T boosters are not regulated by the FDA, and questions remain as to their efficacy and potential mechanisms of action, as most have not been closely studied. The few available controlled studies failed to find an increase in testosterone levels associated with their use, or any improvement in strength. From a fertility standpoint, if they really did enhance endogenous testosterone production, then there should be no detrimental impact on sperm production. However, I recommend that men who are trying to optimize their fertility stop taking T boosters, for two reasons: (1) their production is not regulated by the FDA, so quality control and review of actual ingredients are not under any supervision, and (2) their mechanism of action has not been carefully studied, and therefore certain T boosters may actually have negative hormonal effects on male fertility. For example, ginseng has been shown to contain phytoestrogens, which have female hormonal activity.

Fertility Management of Men Taking Exogenous Androgens

As mentioned earlier, most men taking stronger exogenous androgens—prescription testosterone, anabolic steroids, and some prohormones—see their sperm count drop significantly (oligospermia), and often go to zero (azoospermia), after taking these substances for only three to six months. When they stop taking exogenous androgens, most men will have sperm production return. In some men this may happen as little as three months after the exogenous androgens are stopped, but normally it takes four to six months before sperm production resumes, and it can even take two to three years or longer in some circumstances. Some men never regain their prior sperm production capacity, and a minority (5 percent or so) can remain permanently azoospermic. Factors that affect the speed and degree of sperm production recovery include the type and strength of exogenous androgens used, the length of time they were used, and each person's individual physiologic response. For example, men using transdermal testosterone preparations (patches, gel) tend to require a longer sperm recovery time than men taking testosterone injections.

Men who stop taking exogenous androgens typically experience subsequent low testosterone levels. This can be because their baseline T levels are low (which is why they started taking the androgens in the first place), because their body's endogenous T production remains suppressed even after going off the exogenous androgens, or both. These men therefore frequently need to be started on medications that increase endogenous testosterone production (such as clomiphene, anastrazole, or HCG), both to improve the hormonal environment for sperm production as well as to decrease the adverse symptoms of low testosterone, such as low energy levels and low libido.

I have found that if a man does not feel terrible after stopping his exogenous testosterone, then he is more likely to continue with the recommended treatment plan to maximize his fertility. That's why I will often prescribe medications that increase endogenous testosterone production at the same time that the exogenous androgens are stopped. I usually recommend starting with either a higher dose of clomiphene (50 mg daily) or HCG (2000 IU three times per week) and let the patient make the choice between which of these he wants to start with. Clomiphene is cheaper and can be taken by mouth, but it may not increase the testosterone levels quite as much as HCG. HCG involves injections three times a week and is more expensive than clomiphene. Some men do well on just clomiphene, but a substantial majority will need to be switched over to HCG, and they may feel the effects of low testosterone (low energy, etc.) before they make the switch. I typically repeat a hormone profile two weeks after starting a medication or changing doses, and adjust the medications and dosages as necessary, while also taking into consideration the patient's symptoms. I check a semen analysis three months after the hormone levels have normalized.

For detailed information on endogenous testosterone replacement therapy, see Chapter 7.

Can Men Who Want to Have Children Ever Take Exogenous Androgens?

In couples where the man has stopped taking exogenous androgens and the wife becomes pregnant, a common question is whether he can restart taking exogenous androgens if they want to have more children in the future. Emerging scientific evidence suggests that he should stay off all exogenous androgens while he is still interested in conceiving children. When men use exogenous androgens intermittently, their sperm production typically rebounds each time they are "off cycle"—but often sperm numbers and quality do not recover to the same baseline levels that they had prior to restarting the exogenous androgens. This progressive decrease in sperm quality can impair a couple's future fertility chances, so it is best to stick with increased endogenous production alone until the couple's fertility efforts are complete.

Some men are very reluctant to stop exogenous testosterone therapy (for example, professional bodybuilders). I think that if the couple really wants the best chance of conceiving a child, then the man should stop taking exogenous androgens and switch over to medications that increase endogenous T production. However, for men who refuse to stop taking anabolic steroids or other exogenous androgens, there have been some studies that show that being on low-dose HCG at the same time as exogenous androgens may somewhat protect sperm production.

In one study, men were given exogenous testosterone by injection or gel, as well as low-dose HCG injections (500 IU three times per week). The study found that these men were able to maintain elevated intra-testicular testosterone levels on this regimen. Semen parameters were decreased, but no men experienced azoospermia.* Again, these results are preliminary, and clearly sperm counts would likely be optimized by stopping all exogenous androgens, but this type of combined regimen is a potential option for some men who wish to preserve some degree of fertility despite using exogenous androgens.

* T. C. Hsieh, A. W. Pastuszak, K. Hwang, and L. I. Lipshultz, "Concomitant Intramuscular Human Chorionic Gonadotropin Preserves Spermatogenesis in Men Undergoing Testosterone Replacement Therapy," *Journal of Urology* 189, no. 2 (February 2013).

Glossary of Fertility-Related Medical Problems

The following is a list (in alphabetical order) of medical problems that can be associated with decreased male fertility. This is not a complete list, but it does address some of the more common fertility-related general medical problems.

Androgen Insensitivity Syndrome (AIS)

Men with AIS have problems with their androgen receptors and therefore the cells of their body do not recognize testosterone. Since their cells cannot bind to and utilize testosterone, these men suffer from severe hypogonadism despite very high levels of testosterone in their bloodstreams. The physical characteristics of these men depend on the severity of the abnormalities of their androgen receptors. In complete AIS, there is no testosterone action at all in the cells. Though genetically male, these patients are born with female genitalia at birth and look like females, though they have no internal female sex organs. In men with partial AIS, there remains some level of testosterone action in the cells. Therefore these men can have some development of male genitalia, ranging from partial development to normal development. On blood testing, these men have elevated levels of LH and testosterone. Depending on the severity of the receptor defect, men with partial AIS can have fertility issues ranging from mild sperm abnormalities to complete azoospermia.

Beta-thalassemia

Beta-thalassemia involves a problem with normal hemoglobin synthesis (hemoglobin carries oxygen in the blood). Men with this problem require repeat blood transfusions over their lifetimes. These blood transfusions can result in a buildup of iron deposits within different parts of the body. If enough iron builds up within the pituitary gland, this can decrease FSH and LH release. Iron deposits within the testicles can also lead to testicular failure.

Cancer Treatment

Cancer treatments are designed to kill cells that are rapidly dividing, as cancer cells usually are. Unfortunately, the spermato-genic cells that form sperm also divide quickly, and therefore are often damaged or killed during the course of cancer treatments. Most patients who receive chemotherapy and/or pelvic radiation experience severe decreases in sperm production, with the severity of the effect dependent upon the type of therapy received. The majority of these patients eventually recover some degree of sperm production, although approximately 25 percent remain azoosper-mic permanently.

In addition to the decreases in sperm count and quality, studies have found temporary genetic changes in sperm following chemo-therapy and radiation therapy, with the potential for an increased risk of fetal abnormalities. It is therefore recommended that men wait anywhere from six to twenty-four months following chemo-therapy or radiation therapy before using ejaculated sperm for reproduction (ask your oncologist for specific recommendations on how long to wait, as the recommended times may differ depending on which type of treatment or agents you received, as well as situational factors related to your cancer). Sperm DNA fragmentation as well as sperm FISH (fluorescent in situ hybridization) testing is sometimes used to evaluate the genetic quality of sperm that has returned in the first few years after completing cancer therapy (see Chapter 11 for more details on advanced sperm testing).

Men who may want to have children in the future should bank (freeze) sperm prior to starting chemotherapy or radiation therapy. It's best to bank sperm before the start of cancer treatment, if at all possible, as once radiation or chemotherapy has started, genetic changes can be found in sperm.

Sometimes the stress on the body from fighting cancer cells can decrease sperm counts and quality even before any chemotherapy or radiation therapy has taken place. In certain cases, men with a new diagnosis of cancer do not have any sperm in their ejaculate even before starting cancer treatments, and therefore unfortunately have nothing to freeze.

Chemotherapy

Most chemotherapeutic agents have a negative impact on sperm production, with significant decreases in sperm density seen one to two months following the beginning of cancer treatment. The chances of sperm returning to the ejaculate depend on the impact of the chemotherapy on the spermatogenic stem cells: some forms of chemotherapy temporarily suppress the production of sperm from the stem cells, while others tend to kill the stem cells outright. If the stem cells are not killed by the chemotherapeutic agents, then recovery of sperm production usually starts around twelve weeks after finishing the last cancer treatments. This recovery can be delayed in some men, who need two to five years or longer—up to ten years in some patients. If sperm return following chemotherapy, sometimes the semen parameters return to baseline normal, but a significant proportion of men have permanent decreases in sperm density and quality. Some men never have sperm return following completion of chemotherapy. In these persistently azoospermic men, sperm can sometimes be found surgically, for use with IVF/ICSI (see Chapter 9).

Different types of chemotherapy each have their own specific degrees of toxicity to sperm production. The following is an (incomplete) list of chemotherapeutic agents that have been known to have the capacity to kill spermatogenic stem cells, resulting in permanent azoospermia in some men:

- Alkylating agents (chlorambucil, nitrogen mustard, cyclo-phosphamide, procarbazine, melphalan, busulfan, ifosfamide, nitrosoureas)
- Platinum agents (cisplatin, carboplatin, oxaliplatin, etc.)

The following agents typically result in temporary decreases in sperm production by themselves. However, if they are used in combination with alkylating or platinum-based agents, they can increase stem cell toxicity even more:

- Adriamycin
- Thiotepa
- Vinblastine
- Cytosine
- Arabinoside

The following agents typically result in temporary decreases in sperm production, and generally do *not* increase stem cell toxicity when used in combination with alkylating or platinum-based agents:

- Mitoxantrone

- Methotrexate

- Dacarbazine

- 5-fluorouracil

- Vincristine

- Taxanes

- Bleomycin

Biologically Targeted Agents

Many newer pharmacologic agents are being developed to treat cancer that work differently than the standard cytotoxic chemo drugs. There's limited information about the impact of these newer agents on male fertility, but preliminary data indicate that most biological agents have minimal effects on sperm numbers and quality (there are a few exceptions, described below). The most common fertility-related impact seen with biological agents involves changes in hormone levels.

Examples of biological agents and their currently known fertility impacts include:

- *Tyrosine kinase inhibitors, such as imatibinib (Gleevec), sunitinib, and dasatinib.* These drugs have modest or no impact on spermatogenesis, though they can decrease testosterone levels and cause gynecomastia (breast enlargement) in some patients.

- *Interferon alpha.* No significant impact on male fertility has been noted.

- *Immunomodulating agents, such as alemtuzumab (Campath).* No significant impact on sperm production has been seen, though they may cause reversible agglutination of sperm after around three months.

- *mTOR inhibitors, such as rapamycin and sirolimus.* There is some evidence they may decrease sperm counts and testosterone levels.

- *Targeted radionuclides.* These deliver radiation to certain tissues, and they can decrease sperm production if testicular tissue is affected.

Radiation Therapy

Radiation therapy is a type of treatment for cancer that uses ionizing radiation to kill rapidly dividing cancer cells. The impact of radiation therapy on spermatogenic stem cells depends on where the radiation is targeted. Head and neck radiation would be expected to have a negligible impact on sperm production, as opposed to radiation therapy to the pelvis. When the testicles do receive radiation at high enough dosages, sperm counts typically experience a rapid decline starting about ten weeks after the radiation begins. Complete azoospermia is typically seen at around eighteen weeks after therapy begins. Some men can experience permanent azoospermia depending on the testicular dosage received. In some circumstances, testosterone levels can also be decreased because of damage to the Leydig cells.

Another distinctive characteristic of radiation is that tissue damage can evolve and worsen over the course of years in some people. So in contrast with chemotherapy, in which the semen parameters immediately worsen and then typically improve, semen parameters following radiation therapy can continue to worsen over time in some men. As with chemotherapy, it is generally not recommended to use ejaculated or extracted sperm for at least six to twenty-four months following the conclusion of radiation therapy, because of the potential for damage to the sperm's DNA; this could theoretically increase the chance of birth defects in the offspring.

Prostate brachytherapy is a form of therapy in which small radioactive seeds are placed directly into the prostate gland to treat prostate cancer. Short-term studies do not show a significant change in semen parameters at six months. However, studies with longer follow-up have found significant decreases in sperm counts and quality as well as increases in sperm DNA fragmentation up to four years and longer following brachytherapy. Radiation therapy of the prostate (with brachytherapy or with external beam radiation) can also affect the ability of the prostate and seminal vesicles to produce the healthy semen fluid that is needed for successful natural fertility.

Celiac Disease

Celiac disease is an autoimmune disease of the small intestine. Symptoms including abdominal pain, diarrhea, constipation, and fatigue can occur if someone with celiac disease consumes gluten, a protein found in wheat and a number of other grains. Some men with celiac disease have been reported to have increased levels of androgen resistance, in which the body's cells are not as responsive to testosterone as they should be; this can potentially lead to abnormalities of semen parameters. There is some evidence that these negative hormonal and fertility effects can be improved with avoidance of gluten containing foods.

Chemotherapy

See "Cancer Treatment," above.

Ciliary Diseases

Cilia are small hair-like structures commonly found in the respiratory tract, where they help sweep out foreign objects and bacteria that are inhaled. Cilia also form the tails of sperm, providing them with the ability to swim. There are several genetic abnormalities that can impair the ability of the cilia to move properly, resulting in sperm that are alive, but cannot swim. These include immotile cilia syndrome and Kartagener's syndrome.

In immotile cilia syndrome (ICS), the cilia do not work properly, and therefore people with this disease have chronic respiratory infections due to an inability to effectively clear mucus, bacteria, and foreign objects from the lungs. Cilia are also found in the sinuses and middle ear, so these patients often suffer from chronic sinusitis. Men with ICS are typically infertile, as the tails of the sperm do not function. The sperm are alive but cannot swim up the fallopian tubes to fertilize any eggs. The diagnosis can be made with special testing called electron microscopy (which is not widely available outside of large research universities). Pregnancy can be achieved using the sperm in conjunction with IVF/ICSI.

Kartagener's syndrome is a form of ICS in which the man also has situs inversus, a condition in which the locations of the major organs are reversed within the body (i.e., the heart is located on the right side of the body instead of the left). This reversal of organs typically does not have any significant health implications.

Cirrhosis/Liver Disease

Men with liver disease have higher rates of:

- Hypogonadism
- Elevated estradiol levels
- Testicular atrophy
- Erectile dysfunction
- Gynecomastia (breast enlargement)

Congenital Adrenal Hyperplasia (CAH)

CAH involves a genetic abnormality that disrupts the ability of the adrenal glands to make cortisol. In normal circumstances, the adrenal glands also produce about 10–20 percent of the androgens in the body. In men with CAH, the substances that usually serve to make cortisol are instead converted into elevated levels of androgens. Men with CAH typically have early onset of puberty due to the higher than normal circulating levels of androgens. In adulthood, these elevated levels of adrenal androgens have a negative feedback effect on the pituitary gland, resulting in suppression of FSH and LH production. This has a predictable negative impact on sperm production. Milder variants of CAH can also be present, in which cortisol production is only partially blocked; these men typically develop milder symptoms later in life.

The diagnosis of CAH usually involves blood testing for adrenal-related abnormalities, including:

- Elevated 17-OHP (normal: $31-220$ ng/dL)
- Elevated ACTH (normal 9–52 pg/mL)
- Elevated androstenedione (normal: 60–270 ng/dL)

Adrenal imaging should also be performed to rule out the presence of an adrenal tumor as the source of elevated blood androgens.

From a fertility standpoint, men with CAH typically present with low sperm count (oligospermia) or a zero sperm count (azoospermia), low FSH levels, testicular atrophy, and high testosterone levels. Benign testicular rest tumors are present in 25–50 percent of men with CAH, and these can cause local testicular damage or obstruction in some cases. Treatment of CAH involves cortisol replacement, typically in the form of dexamethasone. Effective treatment of CAH can reverse the adverse fertility hormone profile and restore fertility in some men. The benign testicular rest tumors can also shrink or disappear when the CAH is successfully treated.

Crohn's Disease

Crohn's disease is a type of inflammatory bowel disease that can lead to nutrient deficiencies. A deficiency of zinc can lead to fertility issues in some men with Crohn's disease.

Cryptorchidism

Cryptorchidism is a term used to describe the condition of having undescended testicles, in which one or both testicles have not dropped down into the scrotum by the time of birth. This occurs in approximately 3–5 percent of full-term babies, with higher rates in premature infants. By one year of age, the testicles will have spontaneously descended into their normal position in the scrotum in 75 percent of full-term and 95 percent of premature infants born with cryptorchidism.

From a fertility perspective, the normal position of the testicles within the scrotum allows them to remain two to three degrees cooler than the rest of the body. When the testicles remain stuck in the inguinal region or abdomen, their environment is much warmer than it should be. This typically results in permanent damage to the testicles if they are not brought down into the scrotum in a timely manner. The higher the testicle position within the body, the higher the temperature and thus the greater the potential damage to the testicle.

Studies have shown that testicular spermatogenic cells usually do not suffer any irreversible damage if the testicles come down into the scrotum between six and fifteen months of age. By two years of age, however, 30 percent of undescended testicles have suffered permanent damage, and this percentage increases further with advancing age. The American Academy of Pediatrics recommends treatment for cryptorchidism if the testicle has not descended on its own by the time a child has reached one year of age. Surgical treatment involves orchidopexy (also called orchiopexy), in which the testicle is brought down into the scrotum and fixed in this position with permanent sutures.

Semen abnormalities are found in 20–75 percent of men with one undescended testicle (and 50–90 percent of men with two undescended testicles) who received delayed treatment or no treatment.

Other problems associated with cryptorchidism include:

- Increased risk of congenital epididymal abnormalities (such as obstruction)
- Increased risk of testicular cancer (thus I recommend that men who had an undescended testicle do regular self-exams for testicular lumps, with ultrasound evaluation of any lump found)
- Increased risk of testicular torsion
- Increased risk of developing an inguinal hernia

Diabetes

Diabetes is a common cause of neurologic and vascular damage, because of to the negative impact of persistently elevated blood sugars on the body's nerves and blood vessels. The influence of diabetes on ejaculation and erectile function depends upon the degree of neurologic and vascular injury, and can take one or more of several forms, including:

- Retrograde ejaculation (from incomplete closing of the bladder neck)
- Anejaculation (from paralysis of reproductive tract smooth muscle, which has been replaced by fibrotic tissue)
- Failure of emission (sperm are not deposited into the ure-thra)

- Erectile dysfunction (affects approximately 35–75 percent of men with type 1 diabetes)
- Calcification of the seminal vesicles (makes them unable to contract and propel sperm into the urethra; electroejaculation does not work well in these patients)

See the "Erectile Dysfunction" and "Ejaculatory Problems" sections of this chapter for more detailed information.

Epididymitis

Inflammation or infection of the epididymis (epididymitis) is a relatively common finding in young men. Symptoms can range from none at all to severe scrotal pain (which can mimic testicular torsion). Epididymitis can be caused by an infection as well as by non-infectious inflammation; the latter is more common in men trying to conceive. In older men, the most common cause of infectious epididymitis is E. coli bacteria, while in men under thirty-five, the most common causes are sexually transmitted diseases such as chlamydia and gonorrhea. Epididymitis can lead to pyospermia, which can have a negative impact on sperm numbers and quality (see "Elevated White Blood Cells (Pyospermia)" earlier in this chapter).

Risk factors for non-infectious epididymitis include:

- Lifting heavy objects
- Travel that includes prolonged periods of sitting
- Bike/motorcycle riding

Glucocorticoid Excess

Glucocorticoids are steroid hormones made naturally by the body in the adrenal glands. Too high a level of glucocorticoids in the body can potentially lead to a decrease in LH in some men, which can lead to hypogonadism and an abnormal semen analyses. Excess glucocorticoids can occur because corticosteroid medications (such as prednisone) have been taken for extended periods of time, or because of Cushing's disease, in which the body is producing too many of its own corticosteroids

Hemochromatosis

Hemochromatosis is a genetic abnormality involving dysregulation of the absorption of iron. The resulting iron overload can cause abnormal deposits of iron to build up in the pituitary gland and testicles. If enough iron accumulates in the pituitary gland, FSH and LH release can be impaired. Excessive iron deposits within the testicles can also lead to testicular failure.

Hypospadias

Hypospadias is a congenital problem characterized by an abnormal location of the meatus (the opening on the penis). Mild cases of hypospadias, in which the opening is still near the tip of the penis, do not typically impact male fertility significantly. However, if the meatus is not near the tip of the penis, then the sperm are not deposited close to the cervix during intercourse and ejaculation. Most cases of severe hypospadias in the United States are identified and corrected during early childhood. Persistent problems in adulthood can be corrected surgically, or the problem can be bypassed by using sperm collection combined with intrauterine insemination.

Inguinal Hernia Repair

The vas deferens and blood supply of the testicles pass through the inguinal canal on their way to the scrotum. During repair of an inguinal hernia, these structures can be inadvertently damaged, with the risk being higher in hernia repairs during childhood, when these structures are significantly smaller. The risk of damaging the vas deferens during an inguinal hernia repair in adults is about 1–2 percent, with somewhat higher rates for repeat hernia repairs and repairs in children. The risk of significantly damaging the blood supply to the testicle during a hernia repair is generally felt to be around 1 percent.

About 3–4 percent of men who have had an inguinal hernia repair also have ejaculatory dysfunction (see "Ejaculatory Problems" later in this chapter). The cause is not completely clear, but one idea is that the mesh that has been placed in the body during the repair process causes nerve entrapment. The resulting nerve inflammation and irritation can cause pain during sexual intercourse and ejaculation, leading to ejaculatory disorders. Potential treatments include careful mesh incision and transection of the ilioinguinal and iliohypogastric nerves by a pain specialist, if conservative treatments (such as corticosteroid or local anesthetic injections into the area) have not been effective.

Myelodysplasia/Spina Bifida

Congenital abnormalities of the developing neural tube during fetal development can result in the abnormal formation of some of the vertebral bodies that normally protect the spinal cord. Depending on the severity of the defect, varying amounts of the spinal cord contents may protrude out of the vertebral body, resulting in permanent neurologic damage. This nerve damage can lead to varying degrees of erectile and ejaculatory problems in some men.

Myotonic Dystrophy

Myotonic dystrophy is a progressive disease characterized by muscle wasting, heart problems, cataracts, and hormone abnormalities. Eighty percent of men with muscular dystrophy have significant testicular atrophy and sperm production problems.

Orchitis/Mumps

Orchitis is inflammation and/or infection of the testicles. Inflammation in this area can be caused by bacteria, viruses, or non-infectious causes. Orchitis can be a source of pyospermia (although epididymitis and prostatitis are more common causes of pyospermia). Orchitis is typically painful, but in some men it can be a chronic, asymptomatic problem.

Mumps is the most common cause of viral orchitis. Orchitis develops in about 20–30 percent of men who contract mumps after puberty, and one in ten of these cases involves both testicles. Intense swelling and inflammatory changes can accompany the orchitis, and typically cause significant scrotal pain. If not managed with early high-dose corticosteroids or interferon, mumps orchitis often results in permanent damage to the testicle, which can atrophy and become nonfunctional. The atrophic changes typically occur within the first six months, but sometimes they can take years to develop. In men with untreated mumps orchitis, approximately 10–15 percent will have fertility problems if only one testicle was affected, and 30–90 percent if both testicles were involved.

Other viruses that are known to sometimes cause orchitis include echovirus, group B arbovirus, and Epstein-Barr virus (mononucleosis).

Pituitary Insufficiency (Hypopituitarism)

The pituitary gland is the major hormone control center of the brain. Pituitary function can be diminished for a number of reasons, including tumors, infections or inflammation, vascular injury, radiation, trauma, and surgery. Various congenital problems (such as Kallman's syndrome—see Chapter 10) can also severely impact the pituitary's function. Follicle-stimulating hormone (FSH), luteinizing hormone (LH), thyroid-stimulating hormone (TSH), adrenocorticotropic hormone (ACTH), growth hormone (GH), and prolactin can all be affected by pituitary gland problems. Symptoms depend on the clinical situation and on which hormone levels are impacted. Tumors in the region of the pituitary gland can be completely asymptomatic, or they can cause symptoms such as headaches and vision changes.

Polycystic Kidney Disease

Polycystic kidney disease is a genetic abnormality that involves extensive cystic changes within the kidneys. These cystic changes can also be seen in the seminal vesicles, which can impact their ability to contract during ejaculation. Mild cases can sometimes be managed with intercourse once or twice a day during the woman's fertile phase. In more severe cases, no fluid is transported through the ejaculatory ducts, and sperm extraction must be employed in order to retrieve sperm for IVF/ICSI (see "Management of Obstructive Azoospermia" in Chapter 9).

Posterior Urethral Valves

Infants may sometimes have abnormal flaps of tissue in the urethra, which result in obstruction of the flow of urine. If left untreated, these posterior urethral valves can lead to urinary retention, recurrent urinary tract infections, abnormal reflux of urine from the bladder back up the ureters, and kidney damage and/or failure. Treatment of posterior urethra valves typically involve resection of the valves through a small scope placed up through the penis.

Approximately 50 percent of men with a history of posterior urethral valves have abnormalities of their semen parameters. About 40 percent of these men report a lack of forceful ejaculation. Some also experience retrograde ejaculation into a dilated posterior urethra area. About 10–15 percent of these patients also have a history of undescended testicles at birth.

Prader-Willi Syndrome

This abnormality is caused by a genetic abnormality on chromosome 15 and is characterized by obesity and mental retardation, among other findings. Pituitary gland hypofunction is common in these patients, resulting in significant hypogonadism.

Prostatitis

Inflammation of the prostate is something urologists see relatively often. Symptoms can range from none (the most common situation) to severe irritation when urinating (similar to a urinary tract infection). Most cases of prostatitis in young men are due to non-infectious inflammation; however, bacteria are the cause of the problem in up to 10–20 percent of cases. Prostatitis can cause male fertility problems due to the presence of pyospermia (see "Elevated White Blood Cells (Pyospermia)" earlier in this chapter).

Prune Belly Syndrome

Prune belly syndrome is a genetic abnormality resulting in lax abdominal muscles, along with bilateral undescended testicles and a small, underdeveloped prostate gland. Abnormal development of the vas deferens, seminal vesicles, and epididymis is also common. There are no documented cases of men with this syndrome achieving successful pregnancies by natural intercourse, but extracted sperm have been used successfully in combination with IVF/ICSI. As with most genetic diseases, genetic counseling is strongly recommended prior to fertility treatments to discuss the potential risk of transmitting this condition to offspring.

Radiation Therapy

See the "Cancer Treatment" section earlier in this chapter.

Renal Failure

Decreases in kidney function can cause the following problems, all of which may have a negative impact on fertility:

- Nutritional deficiencies
- Elevated estradiol
- Elevated prolactin
- Low testosterone
- Decreased libido
- Erectile dysfunction

Hemodialysis, used to treat kidney failure, itself has been associated with decreased levels of testosterone and increased levels of estradiol. Semen parameters have been shown to inversely correlate with the length of time a man has been on dialysis. Kidney transplantation can reverse many of the sexual and fertility abnormalities associated with renal failure and dialysis. Even though immunosuppressive drugs, such as cyclosporine, are known to potentially have a negative impact on semen parameters, they tend to have less of a negative fertility impact on most people than does dialysis.

Retractile Testicles

Retractile testicles are a mild form of undescended testicles in which the cremasteric muscles in the scrotum are hyperactive, thereby drawing the testicles high up within the scrotum for prolonged periods. This has been shown to increase the temperature of the testicles in some men, possibly impacting semen parameters. Some findings have suggested that early surgical treatment could help to avoid problems, although these recommendations have not been confirmed in large studies.

Sarcoidosis

This is a multi-system disease characterized by granulomas (areas of inflammation) in the lungs and throughout the body. The cause is unknown. These granulomas can involve the epididymis in some men, leading to obstructive azoospermia.

Sickle Cell Anemia

This is a genetic abnormality in the body's synthesis of hemoglobin (which carries oxygen in the blood). It causes red blood cells to form an abnormal sickle shape, leading to various complications throughout the body. Sickle cell patients are at an increased risk of experiencing micro-infarcts of the pituitary gland and testicles, thereby damaging their function over time. Repeat blood transfusions can also result in a buildup of iron within the pituitary gland and testicles, causing further damage. Many men with sickle cell anemia therefore often have hypogonadism, testicular atrophy, and abnormal semen analyses.

Spinal Cord Injury

See "Ejaculatory Problems" later in this chapter for more details.

Testicular Cancer

Testicular cancer can cause fertility problems in multiple ways:

- At the time of diagnosis, before any treatment, 50 percent of men with testicular cancer have a low sperm count (oligospermia) and 10 percent have a total absence of sperm (azoospermia). This decrease in sperm production is likely a result of stress on the body as well as a by-product of the immune system's efforts to fight the cancer. Of men who had azoospermia when their cancer was diagnosed, approximately 40 percent will see return of some sperm to the ejaculate after the affected testicle has been removed.

- Orchiectomy (surgical removal of the testicle) is the standard first-line therapy for testicular cancer. Removing one of the testicles can obviously have an impact on future sperm production, although sometimes, as described above, removing the affected testicle can improve sperm count if it was low or zero as a result of the cancer.

- Following orchiectomy, radiation and/or chemotherapy are sometimes necessary to treat or prevent metastatic disease. Both radiation and chemotherapy can have a significant negative impact on sperm production (see "Cancer Treatments," above).

Men who are diagnosed with testicular cancer but would like to have children in the future should always attempt to freeze sperm prior to treatment. If no sperm are present prior to orchiectomy and the patient will need subsequent radiation or chemotherapy, they can try to freeze sperm again after the orchiectomy and before starting radiation or chemo. Ideally, sperm should not be frozen after radiation or chemotherapy has started, due to the potential for those treatments to cause DNA changes in the sperm.

Testicular Torsion

Torsion is a very painful medical problem in which the testicle twists within the scrotum, thereby cutting off its blood supply. This is a medical emergency that requires immediate surgical repair. If the blood supply is not restored to the testicle within six to ten hours, irreversible damage to the testicle often results.

Urethral Stricture Disease

Scar tissue in the urethra typically does not significantly affect the flow of sperm, unless it has progressed to the point where the patient is in complete urinary retention and is emptying his bladder by other means (such as via a suprapubic urinary catheter inserted through the lower abdominal wall). Surgeries to treat urethral stricture disease, however, can result in scar tissue in the area of the verumontanum, resulting in ejaculatory duct obstruction in some men (see "Ejaculatory Problems," below).

Young's Syndrome

Young's syndrome is a rare condition in which the mucus in the respiratory and genital ductal systems is abnormally thick. This results in a triad of symptoms: bronchiectasis (irreversible dilation of lung passages), recurrent sinusitis, and obstructive azoospermia. The thick mucus results in a blockage of sperm transport, typically within the epididymis. Sperm can be extracted surgically and used in conjunction with IVF/ICSI.

Varicoceles

Varicoceles, or abnormally dilated veins in the scrotum, are quite common in the general population, with studies showing them to be present in 5 to 25 percent of all men. Thankfully, the majority of these are not clinically significant. However, they are one of the leading causes of male-factor infertility—about 20 to 40 percent of men with infertility issues have varicoceles.

Several factors can play a role in the development of varicoceles, including the smooth muscle content of the walls of the scrotal veins, how effectively the one-way venous valves are functioning, and increased pressure within the veins (because of their anatomic position).

Most varicoceles are small and do not cause problems with fertility: 80–85 percent of men with varicoceles experience no problems with conceiving children. However, if the veins get large enough, then the pooling of blood in these dilated vessels can interfere with the normal heat exchange mechanisms of the body, which help to keep the testicles two to three degrees cooler than the rest of the body. The resulting elevations in scrotal temperature over time can lead to decreased sperm production and quality, low testosterone levels, decreased testicular size, elevated levels of sperm DNA fragmentation, and increased oxidative stress.

A few important points to remember about varicoceles:

- Varicoceles typically first show up during adolescence. It is possible, in rare circumstances, that certain activities (like extreme powerlifting, which increases intra-abdominal pressures) can increase the chance of developing varicoceles. Typically, however, varicoceles are something that some men were born with a propensity to develop, and they are not a result of lifestyle choices or activities. Varicoceles can occasionally run in families.

- Varicoceles can cause a progressive decrease in sperm counts over time, due to the progressive heat damage. Therefore, varicoceles are the most common cause of what is called secondary infertility. This is where a couple has progressively worsening problems with conceiving children over time.

- Typically the larger the varicocele, the higher the chance of it causing fertility-related problems. Large varicoceles are not always associated with the presence of abnormal semen parameters, although these men are at an increased risk of developing fertility problems with time and should be followed closely if they wish to have further children.

- A varicocele on one side can impact sperm production on both sides.

- Varicoceles that are having a negative effect on sperm production are often associated with decreased testicular volumes on at least one side (although, as noted above, the effect on sperm production can impact both testicles).

- Because of the structure of the venous system, varicoceles are more commonly found on the left side. Approximately 80–90 percent of men with varicoceles have them on the left side only, with the rest having them on both sides. If they are found on both sides (bilateral varicoceles), then the left-sided varicocele is usually larger. If only a large, right-sided varicocele is found, then abdominal imaging (ultrasound or CT scan) should be considered to check for possible masses or variations in venous anatomy.

- Most varicoceles are completely asymptomatic, but in a small minority of patients they can be associated with a dull aching discomfort or a dragging sensation in the scrotum. This discomfort tends to worsen after the man has been on his feet for a while, and improves when he lies down.

Diagnosis of Varicoceles

Size matters with varicoceles. Small varicoceles are typically not considered to be clinically significant, but larger ones can be. Varicoceles are most commonly diagnosed in one of two ways: either by physical examination of the scrotum or by ultrasound imaging. An important rule for diagnosing varicoceles accurately is that the man must be standing position, both for physical exam and for ultrasound evaluation. When a man lies down, the varicoceles tend to collapse, since the downward pressure exerted on them by gravity is decreased.

Physical Exam

With the man standing, the doctor palpates the spermatic cord structures above the testicles in the scrotum, to feel for dilation of the veins. Then the man is typically asked to perform a Valsalva maneuver (it's usually done by closing the mouth and pinching the nose shut, then trying to exhale), which increases the pressure in his abdominal area. If a varicocele is present, this increase in abdominal pressure can typically be felt as an "impulse" or bump against the examiner's fingers, which are around the scrotal veins.

(It is worth noting that every so often, a man can feel light-headed during the scrotal evaluation. This is due to a vasovagal response—essentially, the parasympathetic nerves in the scrotum are activated, causing the veins in the legs to dilate and blood to pool there. If this occurs, the exam should be stopped and the man should lie down. A drink of water and a damp, cold towel on the head often help.)

Varicocele Grading System

Varicoceles are assigned a grade by the physician doing the exam:

Subclinical: the varicocele cannot be felt on physical exam, and is only seen on ultrasound

Grade 1: an impulse can be felt during the Valsalva maneuver, but there are no veins that feel dilated on examination

Grade 2: scrotal veins feel dilated on examination.

Grade 3: scrotal veins are so dilated that they can be seen through the scrotal skin with visual inspection, and typically feel like a "bag of worms" on physical examination

Subclinical and Grade 1 varicoceles are usually not thought to be clinically significant, whereas Grade 2 and 3 varicoceles can adversely affect semen parameters.

Ultrasound

While the man is standing, the scrotal veins are evaluated in two ways. First, the diameter of the largest veins is measured. Second, while the man performs the Valsalva maneuver, the ultrasonographer looks for reversal of blood flow within the scrotal veins (consistent with faulty valve functioning). See Appendix K for a scrotal ultrasound protocol to evaluate for varicoceles.

The classic definition of the presence of a varicocele by ultrasound is a vein 3 mm or greater in diameter that shows reversal of blood flow by Doppler. I personally feel that a vein between 3.0 and 3.5 mm in size is consistent with a subclinical varicocele, one that cannot be felt on physical exam. Since larger varicoceles tend to have a larger impact on fertility, I feel that only dilated veins larger than 3.5 mm in size are likely to be clinically significant. When reversal of flow is seen in these veins with a Valsalva maneuver, it provides further evidence of the presence of a varicocele. Reversed blood flow is sometimes seen in dilated veins that are not of clinically significant size. When a large dilated vein (greater than 3.5 mm in diameter) is seen but the ultrasound shows no reversal of blood flow, I usually consider that to be clinically significant (as long as the vein is not clotted off, or thrombosed). This is because sometimes the Valsalva maneuver is not performed effectively during the ultrasound.

My definition of what I would consider to be a clinically significant varicocele by ultrasound is controversial. Other experts in the field consider any dilated vein 3.0 mm or larger in size that shows reversal of flow with Valsalva a clinically significant varicocele.

Practical Tips for Diagnosing Varicoceles

If you are working with an experienced male fertility expert, then the first step is the physical exam. In my opinion, a physical exam is all you need if there is no palpable varicocele or a grade 1 or grade 3 varicocele.

However, if a grade 2 varicocele is found, then I typically like to have the man get an ultrasound to check its size. Again, this is controversial, with some experts relying only on the physical exam in order to decide whether to treat varicoceles in the grade 2 size range. However, an interesting study published in 2014 found that when multiple urologists performed a physical exam on men with varicoceles, there was a 25 percent discrepancy in the grade of varicocele they thought that patient had. Thus, the grade a varicocele is assigned depends on who is doing the assessment. I prefer to use ultrasound, as I think it provides more objective measurement data for men with midsized varicoceles, helping inform treatment decisions.

If a good physical exam cannot be performed, then I recommend having an ultrasound. Reasons for an inconclusive physical exam include significant discomfort during examination, a vasovagal response (light-headedness) before the evaluation can be completed, and body structure reasons (e.g., a large hydrocele, extreme obesity).

If you are not working with a male fertility expert, then it may be a good idea to get a scrotal ultrasound in order to get objective measurements of any potentially significant dilated scrotal veins.

Should Varicoceles Be Treated?

The treatment of varicoceles is a very controversial topic in the field of infertility. A review of the existing literature will yield a number of articles concluding that treating varicoceles has no impact whatsoever on improving male fertility, and a number of other articles that support treating them. However, it must be remembered that varicoceles have been recognized as a cause of decreased sperm production for hundreds of years, and a large number of studies have been performed over the past fifty years looking at various ways of treating varicoceles. Many of the review articles that have been published include outcomes for varicocele treatment techniques that are outdated and not very effective, or include large numbers of patients who were treated for clinically insignificant (subclinical or grade 1) varicoceles. After evaluating only the latest clinical data, both the American Urological Association and American Society of Reproductive Medicine concluded that treatment of varicoceles should be offered to infertile men with palpable lesions (grade 2 or 3) and abnormalities in their semen parameters. I personally agree that a varicocele repair can play an important role in restoring fertility to some couples, but I also think it is not necessary for the majority of men with varicoceles. I take into account overall semen parameters, the size of the varicocele, the age of the man's partner, and any female-factor fertility issues to see if a varicocele repair is in the couple's best interest from a fertility standpoint.

The minimum requirements to consider treatment of a varicocele include *all* of the following conditions:

- Clinically significant size (grade 2 or 3, or veins larger than 3.5 mm by ultrasound)
- Abnormal semen parameters
- Normal female fertility evaluation, or no irreversible problems

If the semen parameters are completely normal, then in most cases I do not think treatment of a varicocele is indicated. Possible exceptions to this include suspected varicocele-related scrotal pain or abnormal sperm DNA fragmentation (see below).

Another controversial area involves patients with varicoceles who have a sperm morphology abnormality (isolated teratospermia) but normal sperm counts and motility. Since varicoceles seem to have a larger impact on sperm counts and motility, the American Society of Reproductive Medicine's Practice Committee has issued guidelines suggesting that varicoceles of clinically significant size should not be treated in men who have isolated teratospermia.

If a man has abnormal semen parameters and a varicocele of clinically significant size, then there is an approximately 65–70 percent chance of a significant improvement in sperm counts and motility if the varicocele is treated. As a general rule, the larger the size of the varicocele, the higher the chance of seeing improvements with treatment. If a man has a borderline-sized varicocele (for example, 3.5 mm) and associated testicular atrophy on that side, then I typically quote him a 50 percent chance of improved sperm count and motility with varicocele treatment.

A 65 to 70 percent chance of improved sperm count and quality is pretty good, but these statistics must be balanced with a couple of other considerations. One is that the treatment of varicoceles involves an invasive procedure (see below) requiring some degree of anesthesia. The second is that although improvements in semen parameters can be seen as early as three months after the repair is done, in some men it can take six to twelve months to see improvements. The average time is five to seven months.

Because of these factors, several further considerations need to be taken into account when trying to decide whether to repair a varicocele, including:

- *How long a couple has been trying to conceive.* If a couple has been working on trying to have a baby for over a year, they may not want to wait another six to twelve months to see if a varicocele repair is going to work.

- *The age of the woman.* If she is older (approaching forty or beyond), the average five-to-seven-month delay before seeing improvement in semen parameters becomes an even more important consideration.

- *Other treatments the couple is undergoing.* Stress on the body often temporarily decreases sperm production. Thus treatment of a varicocele, which stresses the body, can itself have a temporary negative effect on sperm. This risk of decrease must be taken into account if the couple is currently undergoing treatments such as intrauterine insemination.

- *The baseline semen parameters.* If the sperm density if very low to start with, then treatment of the varicocele may not have a clinically significant impact, even if it is successful. For example, a couple with a very low sperm count may still need IVF despite improvement in the semen parameters.

How Much Improvement Is Typically Seen with a Successful Varicocele Repair

Technically, a successful procedure is described as one that leads to at least a 50 percent increase in sperm count and quality, although I have regularly seen much higher levels of improvement in some men. In general, if the varicocele is larger, then the improvements tend to be larger after repair, though this is not always the case. Review articles report an average overall increase in sperm density of about 10–12 million sperm per cc, an 11 percent improvement in motility, and a variable impact on morphology. However, what we can expect in terms of improvement does tend to correlate with baseline semen parameters. To take an example, I have certainly seen men with a pre-treatment sperm count of 5–10 million sperm per cc improve to over 20 million sperm per cc. However, if a man is starting out with fewer than 1 million sperm per cc, then getting to 5 million sperm per cc after a varicocele repair (at which point the couple would be a candidate for intrauterine insemination; see Appendix D) would be possible but unlikely.

Men with virtual azoospermia typically have a small number of sperm in the ejaculate, less than 100,000 per cc (see "Virtual

Azoospermia" in Chapter 9). Sometimes men with virtual azoo-spermia do not have enough sperm to even comfortably proceed with IVF/ICSI because the lab is concerned that they will not be able to find enough viable sperm to inject all of the eggs; typically 5 to 20 live sperm are needed. In these circumstances, getting enough sperm for intrauterine insemination (IUI) following a varicocele repair is not a reasonable expectation. For men with virtual azoospermia, successful varicocele treatment would be defined as having a great enough improvement in sperm counts to allow for IVF/ICSI.

In complete azoospermia (where there is no sperm in the ejacu-late), repair of a significant varicocele can sometimes result in the return of some sperm to the ejaculate. If no genetic abnormalities are found (such as Y chromosome microdeletion or karyotype abnormalities), then approximately 20 to 30 percent of men can expect small amounts of sperm to return with successful varicocele treatment. Those who do see some sperm return have an average sperm density in the range of 1–2 million sperm per cc, so IVF/ICSI would still need to be used. There is some evidence that even in men who remain azoospermic following a repair of their varicocele, success rates may be increased when using techniques such as microTESE, although this is controversial (see "Management of Non-Obstructive Azoospermia" in Chapter 9 for more information on sperm extraction).

If a man with virtual or complete azoospermia has had a suc-cessful varicocele repair and sees significant improvements in semen parameters, I strongly recommend that he promptly freeze several semen specimens, as for unclear reasons many of these men will eventually go back to having lower (or absent) sperm counts with time. The time it takes for this regression to occur can range from a few months up to several years.

Suggestions for Managing Significant Varicoceles

The decision whether to treat a clinically significant varicocele should be made while looking at the couple as a whole. The first step is to see how much improvement in semen parameters can be made through non-invasive means (e.g., hormonal treatments, lifestyle changes, supplements, etc.). If semen abnormalities are still present following these conservative measures, then the decision about treatment can be made based upon the wishes of the couple as well as the starting sperm count:

- *Virtual azoospermia, azoospermia.* If there are so few sperm that IVF is not even an option, then treating a varicocele is probably a good idea, as long as the couple is able and willing to have IVF (and if genetic testing of the man reveals no genetic abnormalities). The goal would be to get enough sperm to be able to proceed with IVF using ejaculated sperm.

- *Oligospermia with total motile count under 5 million sperm.* With a total motile count of less than 5 million, there are plenty of sperm for IVF but not enough to be useful for IUI. If the couple would like to avoid IVF if possible and wants to pursue IUI, then treatment of the varicocele would be reasonable. Another approach for a couple that has been trying to conceive for a long time (and wants more than one child) is to proceed with IVF now, and once the woman is pregnant and through her first trimester, then the man could get his varicocele repaired. If it takes six to twelve months to see full improvement, that is not a problem, since the woman will be pregnant through most of that time, and potentially the next child could then be conceived through IUI or natural intercourse.

- *Oligospermia with total motile count over 5 million sperm.* With a slightly higher count, this can be a tough decision. If immediate IUI is successful, then treatment of the varicocele may not be necessary. However, IUI has a higher chance of success with increased sperm count and quality—but it can take six to twelve months to see that improvement, with a 30 to 35 percent chance that the couple waits that long and no improvement even occurs. There is no correct answer here. Some couples choose to proceed with a few cycles of IUI, and if these are not successful, then they proceed with varicocele treatment (or IVF). Again, once the woman is pregnant, elective varicocele repair can be undertaken if the couple wants more children, in the hopes that the next child may be conceived naturally or more easily.

Insurance Coverage of Varicocele Repairs

Varicocele repairs are one of the few fertility treatments that are often (but not always) covered by insurance. Of course, regulations for coverage vary from state to state, as well as between different insurance companies and policies. Check with your insurance company prior to proceeding with treatment.

Diagnosis codes that can be used for varicocele treatment:

Diagnosis	ICD-9 code (before Oct. 2015)	ICD-10 (Oct. 2015 and later)
Varicocele	456.4	I86.1
Testicular atrophy	608.3	N50.0
Scrotal pain	608.9	N50.9 and R10.2

Surgery procedure codes that can be used for varicocele treatment:

Varicocelectomy: 55530

Use of operating microscope: 69990

Embolization procedure codes that can be used for varicocele treatment:

Vascular catheter placement: 36011 and 36012

Vascular embolization for varicocele: 37241

Note that in some states insurance coverage for fertility is limited, but treatment of varicoceles for scrotal pain is often covered.

Management of Future Fertility if a Varicocele Is Not Treated

Many couples will achieve a pregnancy (either naturally or through IUI or IVF) without treating a clinically significant varicocele. If the couple would like to have more children in the future, they have the option of either treating the varicocele while the woman is pregnant or just observing the varicocele. The potential advantage of treating the varicocele electively while the woman is pregnant is that the next pregnancy might be easier to establish. However, given that a pregnancy was achieved the first time, the varicocele might not need to be treated. One point to consider regarding untreated varicoceles is that varicoceles can be associated with a progressive decrease in sperm counts and quality over time. I therefore recommend that when a man with a significant varicocele wants more children, he should get at least a yearly semen analysis to make sure that his numbers are not decreasing significantly over time.

Treatment Options for Varicoceles

There are two main techniques for treating varicoceles: surgical repair (varicocelectomy) and embolization (clotting the veins off using a minimally invasive approach).

Surgical Repair

The goal of varicocelectomy surgery is to tie off or clip the dilated veins, which then scar down over time. The remaining smaller, non-dilated surrounding veins effectively drain away the blood from the testicles, so there is no concern about blocking all blood flow from the scrotum. A few keys to successful surgery include:

- *Adequate visualization of the veins.* Ideally, an operating microscope is used to minimize the chance that significant veins are missed, which can increase the risk that the varicocele will persist or recur.

- *Preservation of the arterial blood supply.* Only veins should be ligated (that is, clipped or tied). It is very important that the arterial blood supply of the testicle be maintained, or else testicular damage and atrophy can occur. The use of an intraoperative Doppler probe can effectively distinguish which vessels are veins and which are arteries.

- *Preservation of the vas deferens.* This structure must be carefully identified and not damaged, as it carries the sperm from the testicle to the penis.

- *Preservation of lymphatic vessels.* These small, delicate vessels have a characteristic translucent appearance under the operating microscope. Lymphatic channels should be preserved to decrease the risk of developing a significant hydrocele (a collection of fluid around the testicle that might require surgical drainage if it gets large enough).

Microscopic Inguinal or Subinguinal Varicocelectomy

The best surgical technique for treating varicoceles in adults is the inguinal or subinguinal microscopic varicocelectomy. In this technique, the spermatic cord (which contains the dilated veins) is approached through a small incision in the inguinal (groin) area.

The inguinal ring is where the spermatic cord emerges from the abdomen into the scrotum. Incisions placed either at the inguinal ring (inguinal) or just below the ring (subinguinal) are effective, providing good access to the various veins that can branch off from the main testicular veins in this area. The inguinal approach tends to be associated with somewhat increased pain and longer recovery times, as opposed to the subinguinal technique. In both approaches, the dilated veins are identified and either tied off with permanent sutures or ligated with surgical clips, while the vas deferens, lymphatic channels, and arteries are identified and preserved.

Varicocelectomy procedures are considered minor surgery, and are typically performed under general anesthesia on an outpatient basis. Most people are off work for five to seven days, though this period of time may be shorter for people with exclusively desk jobs, or longer for people whose jobs require more strenuous activity (construction, law enforcement, firefighting, etc.).

Potential complications of varicocelectomy procedures include:

- *Hydrocele.* A hydrocele—a collection of fluid around the testicle that might require surgical draining—occurs in only 1 percent of cases when microsurgery is employed, versus 7 percent when an operating microscope is not used. Fifty percent of hydroceles grow to a size large enough to eventually require an outpatient surgical treatment for drainage (called hydrocelectomy).

- *Recurrence of the varicocele.* Rates of recurrence of the varicocele in the surrounding veins range from 0 to 35 percent. Lower rates (around 1 to 2 percent) are seen with microscopic techniques using either the subinguinal or inguinal approach.

- *Testicular artery injury.* Seen in approximately 1 percent of cases, this can lead to testicular atrophy and loss of function.

Other Varicocele Surgical Techniques

Several other surgical approaches used for varicocelectomy exist but are not typically used in adults by male fertility specialists. These include:

- *Open retroperitoneal (Ivanessevich) approach.* This is an older surgical technique that accesses the testicular veins higher in the abdominal region. The problem with this approach is that it misses many of the lower venous branch points (external iliac branches) that are found in the inguinal (groin) region. Therefore, rates of persistent or recurrent varicoceles are much higher. These techniques are also typically not performed using operating microscopes, which increases the risk of complications such as hydroceles.

- *Laparascopic approach.* A laparoscope is used to locate and clip off the dilated veins high up in the abdomen near the kidneys. This approach is more common in young children, in whom the inguinal vessels are much smaller and therefore harder to accurately visualize even with an operating microscope (and therefore the risk of arterial blood supply injury is greater). When used in adults, however, the laparoscopic approach has the same drawbacks as the open retroperitoneal approach in that the lower venous (external iliac) branches are not addressed, leading to a potentially higher recurrence rate. Rates of post-procedure hydroceles are low, but the laparoscopic approach through the abdomen does present the small but possible risk of intestinal or major vascular injuries.

Varicocele Embolization

Embolization of varicoceles is a minimally invasive procedure performed by an interventional radiologist (a radiologist who specializes in doing procedures under X-ray imaging guidance). Embolizations are typically performed under IV sedation, in which the patient is made drowsy and essentially sleeps while the procedure is performed. To perform the embolization, the interventional radiologist gains access to the venous system with a needle stick, typically in either the upper leg or neck region. A special small catheter is then placed into the venous system and guided to the area of the dilated veins under X-ray guidance. The dilated veins are then embolized (clotted off), typically using small metal coils or other embolic materials.

The success of embolization must be assessed in three ways:

- *Technical success.* Was the procedure successful in gaining access to the correct veins and effectively clotting them off?
- *Clinical success.* In men in whom the veins were successfully treated, what was the impact on their fertility parameters?
- *Recurrence rate.* What is the rate of varicocele recurrences, which can increase the risk of persistent fertility problems?

Technical Success

The internal spermatic (testicular) veins are the targets of the embolization procedure, and their anatomy differs between the left and right sides. On the left side, the internal spermatic vein typically comes off straight down (at a 90° angle) from the left renal vein, while on the right side the vein comes off at a sharper (more acute) angle from the vena cava, the main large vein that returns blood from the legs and lower body. Because of this sharper angle, the spermatic veins on the right side are more difficult to access than those on the left side. Some radiologists feel that if a neck vein instead of a leg vein is used, the right side might be easier to get access to, coming at it from above instead of from below. Each radiologist has his or her personal preference regarding the best approach to use. In general, however, the rate of failure (that is, failure to gain access) is 3–5 percent on the left side and 15–20 percent on the right side. Most significant varicoceles are on the left, but large right varicoceles may be more difficult to treat with embolization in some cases.

Clinical Success

If the dilated veins are successfully embolized, then success rates in terms of fertility improvement are generally in the same range as those of surgical varicocele repair, with about 65–70 percent of patients experiencing significant improvement in sperm counts and quality.

Recurrence Rates

Rates of recurrence are felt to be higher with embolization than with surgical repair. This, however, does seem to be related to the type of embolization material that is used. Two primary types of techniques can be used: liquid sclerosing agents or specially designed embolic devices.

Sclerosing agents (e.g., sodium tetradecyl sulfate, polydocanol, dextrose solution) are injected into the internal spermatic veins and cause the veins to scar down. Late recurrence rates (significant varicoceles which return after an extended period of time following treatment) with sclerosing agents are 1–2 percent. The advantage of sclerosing agents is that they can be delivered through smaller veins that can be difficult to maneuver a small catheter into. The sclerosing agents can also enter into nearby smaller collateral veins that are connected to the main spermatic veins, thereby causing these smaller vessels to scar down and preventing them from dilating later and resulting in a recurrent varicocele. One disadvantage of sclerosing agents, however, is that they can be associated with more procedure-related discomfort than embolic devices, including thrombophlebitis (vein inflammation related to a blood clot).

There are two primary types of embolic devices, and both have a late recurrence rate of 10 percent. Embolic coils are released into the veins, where they expand and clot off the vein. The clotted-off vein eventually scars down over time. Detachable balloons are released into the veins, where they lodge and cause clotting off of the vein and eventual scar tissue formation.

Complications

The overall complication rate for varicocele embolization is about 10 percent. Most complications are minor, transient, and do not require treatment. However, there are several rare types of serious complications, including those that can result from the sclerosing or embolic agent accidentally traveling to other areas of the body.

Potential complications include:

- Problems with venous access leading to bleeding or damage to nearby structures (less than 1 percent): pneumothorax or mediastinal hematoma with the neck (jugular) approach, and groin hematoma with the leg (femoral) approach
- Severe allergic reactions to the contrast medium used (less than 1 percent)
- Pulmonary embolism due to agent migration (less than 2 percent)
- Renal vein thrombosis (less than 1 percent)
- Testicular atrophy due to thrombophlebitis (less than 1 percent): the risk of this is higher with use of sclerosing agents than with embolic devices

Potential Advantages of Embolization

Compared to surgical repair, embolization has several potential advantages:

- *Minimally invasive procedure.* Embolization involves only venous access (a needle stick) instead of an incision. Therefore, men typically only have to take one or two days off after the procedure instead of the five to seven days necessary with open surgery. They can usually return to full physical activity four to seven days after embolization, compared to two to three weeks with surgery. Generally, men experience a dull ache in the groin or back that last a few days. Less than 5 percent of men undergoing embolization experience more severe pain requiring analgesics or anti-inflammatory medications; if present, this pain can last an average of two days.

- *Less anesthesia needed.* IV sedation is usually adequate for embolization, instead of the full general anesthesia needed for surgery.

- *Potentially faster time to improved semen parameters with a successful procedure.* The minimally invasive embolization procedure is typically associated with less physiologic stress on the body, and there is evidence that in some men sperm counts and sperm quality may rebound faster than with open surgical repair.

- *No risk of damage to the testicular blood supply.* Embolization procedures stay within the venous system, and therefore inadvertent damage to the arterial blood supply of the testicle is not a concern.

Potential Disadvantages of Embolization

Embolization also has some potential disadvantages when compared to surgical repair:

- *Inability to gain adequate venous access.* Due to variations in venous anatomy, about 10 percent of the time (3–5 percent on the left and 15–20 percent on the right), the interventional radiologist cannot get the specially designed catheter to the dilated testicular veins that need to be treated.

- *Recurrence rates.* Rates of recurrent varicoceles can be higher with embolization, as the lower venous channels (external spermatic veins) may not be treated as effectively, especially if sclerosing agents are not used. Overall, with embolization the rates of recurrence are still quite low (1–10 percent), but they are higher than the rates with microsurgical varicocelectomy procedures (1–2 percent).

- Potential migration of embolic material. The chance that a coil, balloon, or sclerosing agent will migrate a significant distance away from where it is inserted is low (less than 1–2 percent), but if this migration occurs, it can have potentially severe consequences. Some people have concerns about coils becoming dislodged and traveling to other parts of the body years down the road. However, the risk for migration is generally present only at the time of the procedure. Once the coils or balloons are in place, the veins scar down, thereby entrapping the clips in the area, so that they generally cannot move.

Optimizing Success with Embolization

One of the keys to success with varicocele embolization is working with an interventional radiologist who routinely performs these procedures. If you are working with a male fertility specialist, he or she should know the names of nearby interventional radiologists who are good at the procedure. Otherwise, you can call a large interventional radiology group and ask them which doctor in their group performs the most varicocele embolization procedures. Ask the interventional radiologist how many varicocele embolizations he or she performs each year. If you live in a fairly big town and the radiologist does at least a few a month, then he or she is probably fairly well experienced. If you work with an interventional radiologist who rarely performs these procedures, you may have a higher chance of an unsuccessful treatment outcome or complications.

Other Potential Health and Fertility Concerns Associated with Varicoceles

Varicoceles and DNA Fragmentation

Clinically significant varicoceles have been associated with elevated levels of DNA fragmentation in some men (see Chapter 11). Varicocele repair has been associated with improvements in sperm DNA fragmentation in up to 90 percent of men, although the degree of improvement was quite modest in most studies. One study showed a 14% improvement in the sperm DNA fragmentation index (DFI) [from 35 percent to 30 percent] in a group of men following varicocele repair, and another showed a 25 percent decrease in DFI by three to six months after the repair.

Varicoceles and Hypogonadism

In addition to changes in their sperm production, men with clinically significant varicoceles have been shown to have lower testosterone levels. In general, the Leydig cells, which make testosterone, are more resistant to damage than the spermatogenic cells, but if the varicocele is large enough, then testosterone levels may be impacted as well. Several studies have shown improvements in testosterone levels in men undergoing varicocele repair for fertility problems. One meta-analysis showed that testosterone levels rose by an average of 87.5 ng/dL following varicocele repair. Another study showed that increases in testosterone were generally higher in men with larger and bilateral varicoceles. For example, in men with bilateral large (grade 3) varicoceles, 86 percent of them showed improvement, with an average testosterone increase of 160 ng/dL. In contrast, in men with only a left-sided, moderate-sized (grade 2) varicocele, 73 percent showed an elevation of testosterone, with an average rise of 103 ng/dL.

It is therefore widely believed that in men with hypogonadism and fertility problems, treatment of a clinically significant varicocele can improve both semen parameters and testosterone levels. However, what remains controversial is the treatment of men with varicoceles who do not have any fertility problems, in an attempt to treat or prevent hypogonadism. A few centers in the country currently treat varicoceles in men with low testosterone and no fertility problems. A potential advantage of this approach is the hope that the man can increase his own endogenous testosterone production and not have to rely on medications to increase testosterone levels.

To date, most urologists do not feel that the scientific evidence is compelling enough to offer invasive varicocele treatment solely for the reason of treating low testosterone levels, although this opinion seems to be slowly evolving with time, with more clinicians considering taking a more aggressive approach.

Erectile Dysfunction

Erectile dysfunction (ED) is a relatively common problem in men being treated for fertility issues. Risk factors include higher rates of hypogonadism (low testosterone), which can affect sperm production as well as erectile function. The psychological stress of trying to coordinate intercourse with a woman's ovulatory cycles can also contribute to a temporary problem with erections in men with fertility issues.

Other risk factors for ED include diabetes, medications (such as beta-blockers, diuretics, and antidepressants), obesity, tobacco use, excessive alcohol use, psychological factors (stress, anxiety, depression), prolonged bicycle riding, and heart disease.

Management of Erectile Dysfunction

The first step in managing ED should include an attempt to decrease or eliminate potentially reversible risk factors, such as cigarette smoking, excessive alcohol use, and prolonged bike riding. Tight blood sugar control can be beneficial in diabetic men, as can gradual weight loss in men with obesity. Stress, anxiety, and depression can be addressed with counseling and/or medications (such as antidepressants, anti-anxiety medications, etc.); however, these psychoactive medications can unfortunately have erectile (and ejaculatory) side effects as well.

Low testosterone levels are a common cause of erectile dysfunction (as well as being a risk factor for abnormal semen parameters). Medications to increase endogenous testosterone production can improve erectile function in men with low testosterone, as well as increase the effectiveness of medications used to treat ED; see Chapter 7.

PDE-5 Inhibitors

PDE-5 inhibitors are oral medications that can help to achieve or sustain an erection longer. Even young, otherwise healthy men often experience temporary erectile problems, especially under the stress of trying to conceive, and in such circumstances PDE-5 inhibitors can help. The use of these medications does not make a man dependent on them in the future for getting erections.

There are four types of PDE-5 inhibitors currently available:

- Sildenafil (Viagra): 50 mg, 100 mg
- Vardenafil (Levitra, Staxyn): 10 mg, 20 mg
- Tadalafil (Cialis): 10mg, 20mg
- Avanafil (Stendra): 50mg, 100mg, 200mg

I do not recommend going above the highest listed doses of these medications, though they can be split into lower dosage pills using a pill cutter. These medications should not be used in combination with each other.

None of these medications will give a man an erection by themselves. Rather, they work by increasing the ability to achieve and sustain an erection with normal sexual stimulation. All of these medications are going to work best if the man has plenty of sexual stimulation, is not rushed or stressed, is well rested, and is in a comfortable environment. There is also evidence that these medications may be more effective if testosterone levels are not lower than normal.

How They Work

Viagra, Levitra, and Staxyn work similarly, in that they are short-acting and achieve maximum blood concentration in about one hour. Therefore, these medications should be taken about an hour prior to anticipated sexual activity. Stendra has a faster time to maximum blood concentration (about fifteen to thirty minutes) and therefore should be taken about fifteen to thirty minutes prior to sexual activity. None of these medications should be taken more than once a day.

Cialis works a little differently in that it needs to be in your system for about an hour before it is effective, but then its blood levels stay elevated for twenty-four to thirty-six hours. (This is not the length of the erection, but rather the time frame for an enhanced ability to achieve and sustain an erection.) Cialis used in this manner should not be taken more than once every other day. Alternatively, Cialis is available in lower doses (2.5mg and 5mg) that can be used daily.

How to Use

It is best to start out with a lower dose of this type of medication and work up to the higher dose as needed. Sometimes multiple trials of a medication are needed before a medication is effective, as men get more comfortable with the medication and the stress of trying something new wears off. Some studies have suggested that a PDE-5 inhibitor should not be considered ineffective unless it has been tried on at least five or six separate occasions. Although none of the PDE-5 inhibitors has been shown to be more effective than any other, sometimes switching to another PDE-5 inhibitor may work if one type is not successful.

Side Effects

Men who stop using PDE-5 inhibitors because of side effects is low, but occasionally bothersome side effects can occur. Sometimes switching to another PDE-5 inhibitor will decrease or eliminate the side effects. Potential side effects include:

- Flushing
- Headache (pre-treatment with acetaminophen or ibuprofen may help)
- Heartburn or acid reflux (consider pre-treatment with antacid medications if this is a problem)
- Nasal congestion
- Temporary blue/green color in vision, or other visual changes

- Back discomfort (primarily seen with Cialis)

Prolonged erections (priapism) that last more than three to four hours are rare with oral PDE-5 inhibitors, but in the event that this happens, the man should be seen in the emergency room as soon as possible. If not treated promptly, priapism can lead to penile damage and scar tissue formation due to a lack of blood flow to the area.

If you experience any severe side effects, stop taking the medication and seek immediate medical help.

Nitrates: Dangerous to Use with PDE-5 Inhibitors

Nitrates are medications that relieve heart disease-related chest pain (angina) by increasing blood flow to the heart. Examples of nitrate medications include Dilatrate, Isordil, Nitro-Dur, Nitrolingual, Nitrostat, and ISMO. Nitrates can also be abused as illegal drugs, and are sometimes called "poppers" (amyl nitrate, butyl nitrite). When used together, PDE-5 inhibitors can have severe negative interactions with nitrates, and can dangerously drop blood pressure to the point of being life-threatening.

Never use PDE-5 inhibitors if you use nitrates. If you have a history of heart disease, chest pain, or nitrate use in the past, or if you need multiple medications to control blood pressure, always get clearance from your primary care doctor or cardiologist before using these medications.

Impact on Fertility

Some small studies have suggested that PDE-5 inhibitors may be detrimental to sperm quality. However, these findings have not been confirmed by larger controlled studies, and I currently do not think that there is much evidence of a significant negative impact on semen parameters. If a man is having trouble even getting his sperm into the female reproductive tract due to erection issues, then this is a much bigger problem than any borderline changes in his sperm quality.

Muse

Muse is the brand name for a small pellet, resembling a grain of rice, that is inserted into the tip of the penis. The medicine (alprostadil) is then absorbed through the urethra into the penis, where it directly increases blood flow, thereby improving erectile function.

Muse should be given for the first time in a doctor's office to assess how a particular man responds to it. Prolonged erections are more common with Muse than with PDE-5 inhibitors, and any erection that lasts more than three to four hours should be promptly evaluated in the emergency room, for if it is left untreated, it can cause irreversible scarring of the penis. Muse is generally considered to be stronger than the PDE-5 inhibitors in the treatment of ED, but less strong than penile injections.

Penile Injections

Biochemically active agents can be injected directly into the penis using a small needle and syringe. Single agents (such as alprostadil) can be injected, as well as combinations of injectable medications (such as Trimix). These medications increase penile blood flow and enhance erectile function. These are the strongest medications for the treatment of ED.

Penile injections should be given for the first time in a doctor's office to assess how a particular man responds to this treatment. Again, prolonged erections are more common with injections than with PDE-5 inhibitors, and any erection that lasts more than three to four hours should be promptly evaluated in the emergency room to avoid irreversible scarring of the penis.

Vacuum Erection Device

Mechanical vacuum erection devices (VEDs) pull blood into the penis, and then an obstructive band is placed around the base of the penis to hold the blood in to maintain an erection. Although these devices can be effective for erections, they are not often used in men of fertility age, as comfort of use and satisfaction rates can be less than ideal. Some men may also experience some blockage of sperm flow with ejaculation due to the compressive ring around the penis.

Couples Sex Therapy

Sometimes couples experience psychological or relationship-related issues that interfere with effectively completing sexual intercourse. This can be a long-standing problem, or it may have developed with the added stress of trying to conceive a child. In these circumstances, working with a well-trained sex therapist can help to both relieve stress and more effectively perform timed intercourse.

For guidance on finding a local sex therapist, consult the website of the American Association of Sexuality Educators, Counselors and Therapists, www.aasect.org.

Ejaculatory Problems

Normal male ejaculation consists of three distinct stages:

1. *Pre-ejaculate.* During erection, prior to reaching orgasm, the bladder neck closes, and the bulbourethral glands (which sit under the prostate gland and open into the urethra) emit a small amount of fluid called pre-ejaculate. This fluid serves to lubricate the urethra as well as to neutralize the acidity of any remaining urine within the urethra, since the acidity can be damaging to sperm.

2. *Emission.* During orgasm, the stimulation of the sympathetic nervous system causes muscular contractions of the vas deferens, thereby carrying the accumulated vasal sperm into the ejaculatory ducts. Contraction of the seminal vesicles causes the seminal vesicle fluid (along with the sperm) to

flow through the ejaculatory ducts and into the urethra, where it mixes with the prostatic fluid.

3. *Ejaculation.* Ejaculation occurs following emission. The rhythmic contraction of the muscles around the base of the penis results in the forceful expulsion of the seminal fluid from the urethra out the tip of the penis. The fluid comes out in a standard order, with the prostatic fluid coming out first, followed by the vasal fluid, and finally the seminal vesicle contents. In young men, this results in a series of rhythmic spurts occurring about 0.8 second apart. As men age into their thirties and forties, they tend to lose this forceful pulsing release of semen, and the fluid come out more slowly (or sometimes just oozes out).

Several types of problems may occur with ejaculation: ejaculatory duct obstruction, retrograde ejaculation, retarded ejaculation, anejaculation, congenital anorgasmia, and painful ejaculation. Each will be discussed below.

Ejaculatory Duct Obstruction

The ejaculatory ducts carry fluid from the seminal vesicles and vas deferens into the urethra. When the ejaculatory ducts are completely blocked, the ejaculate is made up of only the fluid from the prostate. Men with complete ejaculatory duct obstruction (EDO) therefore have the following semen analysis characteristics:

- Low ejaculate volume (less than 1.0 cc), as the fluid from the seminal vesicles and testicles is missing
- A semen pH under 7.2, as prostatic fluid is acidic, and the alkaline seminal vesicle fluid is missing
- No semen fructose, as fructose comes from the seminal vesicles

- Lack of sperm (azoospermia)

EDO is usually completely asymptomatic in men. However, it can sometimes be associated with perineal and/or scrotal pain on ejaculation. It can also be associated with hematospermia (blood in the ejaculate) in some circumstances.

Causes of EDO

EDO can be caused by a number of different problems, including:

- Blockage of the ejaculatory duct by a nearby structure or object, such as a prostatic stone or a cyst (either arising from within the prostate or a cyst left over as a remnant from embryonic development, such as a Mullerian duct cyst)
- Blockage of the ejaculatory duct from scar tissue (such as following urethral surgery, cystoscopy, or insertion of a Foley catheter) or from previous urethral or genital duct infections (such as chlamydia, gonorrhea, or tuberculosis)
- Congenital absence of the ejaculatory duct, such as congenital bilateral absence of the vas deferens (see "Cystic Fibrosis" in Chapter 10).

Partial EDO

The ejaculatory duct can also be partially blocked. The diagnosis of partial EDO can be very tricky, as it can present in a variety of ways. Generally speaking, semen parameters can show any combination of the following, depending on the severity of the blockage:

- Borderline low ejaculatory volume
- Borderline pH
- Decreased motility (often very low)
- Decreased sperm density

- Elevated sperm DNA fragmentation

Possible partial EDO should be suspected in men with border-line ejaculate volumes and very low sperm motility.

Diagnosis of EDO

Men who have azoospermia, low volume, and acidic, fructose-negative ejaculate despite having a normal FSH and normal testicular volume (indicative of likely normal sperm production) are likely not passing any fluid from the seminal vesicles and vas deferens into the urethra. If there is not a palpable vas deferens on each side of the scrotum, then the diagnosis is likely CBAVD (see "Cystic Fibrosis" in Chapter 10). However, if a normal vas deferens can be felt on each side, then there is likely one of two problems present: blockage of the ejaculatory duct (EDO) or acontractile seminal vesicles. With the latter condition, the seminal vesicles cannot contract, which means that fluid may not travel through the ejaculatory ducts into the urethra; the semen analysis is consistent with EDO. Acontractile seminal vesicles are rare, but the condition can result from such problems as advanced diabetes or neurologic abnormalities like a spinal cord injury. Polycystic kidney disease, with large cysts involving the seminal vesicles, can also result in acontractile seminal vesicles. Acontractile seminal vesicles are not generally very responsive to treatment, though the condition may improve if an underlying condition improves (such as neurologic disease).

Using Transrectal Ultrasound (TRUS) for Diagnosis

Transrectal ultrasound (TRUS) involves placing a small ultrasound probe into the rectum. In men with blockage, the ejaculatory ducts and seminal vesicles are often dilated due to a backup of fluid within them.

TRUS measures the following:

- Seminal vesicle diameter (normal is 1.5 cm AP diameter or less)
- Seminal vesicle length (normal is 3 cm or less)
- Ejaculatory duct width (normal is 2 mm, abnormal is 2.3 mm or more)

TRUS can also sometimes show the presence of sources of obstruction, including cysts, calcifications, or masses in the prostate or seminal vesicle. Despite its usefulness, TRUS used by itself has two main drawbacks. One of these drawbacks is that not all EDO patients have dilated seminal vesicles and ejaculatory ducts, though many do. The other is that TRUS cannot differentiate EDO from acontractile seminal vesicles.

Seminal Vesicle Aspiration

In normal circumstances, sperm are not present within the seminal vesicles. However, if fluid is not flowing through the ejaculatory duct normally, then it often backs up into the seminal vesicles, taking sperm with it. At the time of TRUS, a long, narrow needle can be placed under ultrasound guidance into the seminal vesicles and be used to aspirate fluid. The fluid can then be examined microscopically for the presence of sperm. If sperm are present at levels of more than 3 sperm per high power field (hpf) when evaluated with a tabletop microscope, then this suggests possible EDO.

Seminal vesicle aspiration has three limitations:

- If sperm are present in the seminal vesicles, it still does not tell you whether EDO or acontractile seminal vesicles are the problem.

- Some normal, fertile men can have sperm in their seminal vesicles after extended periods of sexual abstinence. A 1996 study found that one-third of normal men have sperm in their seminal vesicles after five days of abstinence (compared to 0 percent at zero days of abstinence).

- Infection risk. When seminal vesicle aspirations are performed, the needle must travel through the rectal wall before entering into the seminal vesicles. Even with a pre-procedure bowel preparation and antibiotics, the rectum is still filled with bacteria, and if these bacteria travel with the needle into a seminal vesicle that is obstructed, then an infection can follow. Since the infection has nowhere to drain, it can potentially form an abscess that may require surgical drainage. However, if the discovered blockage is going to be treated at the same time as needle aspiration (see "TURED," below), then the risk of serious infection is significantly lower, as a successful procedure will involve removing the obstruction and therefore will decrease the risk of an abscess. Studies have not shown this sort of infection to be a major problem; the risk may be more theoretical than actual. However, if a rectal abscess does occur, the consequences can be significant. It is therefore my opinion that if seminal vesicle aspiration is going to be performed, the surgeon should ideally be prepared to perform immediate therapy (for example, TURED) at the same time if the findings are consistent with EDO. This recommendation is controversial, however, with some fertility experts routinely performing diagnostic seminal vesicle aspirations without simultaneous TURED if sperm are found.

Aspirated seminal vesicle sperm (from the blocked seminal vesicles) can potentially be used for IVF/ICSI, but often this does not work very well, since the fluid that is aspirated usually contains large number of old and dead sperm that have accumulated there over time.

Seminal Vesiculography

At the time of TRUS, X-ray contrast media (a special fluid that shows up easily on X-rays) can be injected into the seminal vesicles. A series of X-rays can then be taken to see if this media flows into the urethra and bladder. If the media does make it into the urethra, then EDO is not present (but acontractile seminal vesicles may be present). Enough contrast media needs to be injected so that it is forced to flow through the ejaculatory ducts if no blockage is present.

Chromotubation

Instead of injecting contrast media into the seminal vesicles, chromotubation involves injecting a colored dye (methylene blue or indigo carmine) into the seminal vesicles at the time of TRUS. The patient then undergoes cystoscopy (placing a small scope through the penis) and the doctor looks for the colored dye to come through the ejaculatory ducts into the urethra. Like with seminal vesiculography, if no dye is seen to emerge, then EDO is likely.

A combination of the above procedures can be utilized, in which TRUS is performed and measurements are made of the seminal vesicles and ejaculatory ducts. Seminal vesicle aspiration is performed to check for the presence of sperm. If sperm are seen, then either seminal vesiculography or chromotubation is undertaken in order to differentiate EDO from acontractile seminal vesicles. The whole process takes place at the same time, so if findings consistent with EDO are discovered, TURED can be performed right away (see below).

Vasogram

Another option for diagnosing EDO is vasography. In this proce-dure, a small opening is made in the vas deferens in the scrotum. The vasal fluid is checked for sperm. If sperm are present, then X-ray contrast medium is injected into the vas deferens and X-rays are taken. Similar to seminal vesiculography, if contrast media is seen to flow into the seminal vesicle but not into the urethra or bladder, then EDO is likely present, and TURED can be performed at that time. The risk of vasal scar tissue formation is a drawback of this approach.

Ejaculatory Duct Manometry

A newer form of testing has recently been developed in which the pressures inside the seminal vesicles are measured at the time of TRUS with small pressure-sensitive probes. If EDO is present, then the backup of fluid should increase the pressure within the seminal vesicles. However, if no obstruction is present, then the pressure within the seminal vesicles should be normal. Although promising, this procedure is still in the fairly early stages of use and is of very limited availability.

Treatment of EDO

Sperm Extraction and IVF

Men with EDO typically have normal sperm production (which can be assessed with FSH blood testing). One option is to bypass the obstruction and proceed with sperm extraction combined with IVF/ICSI (see Chapter 9). This approach avoids the need for TURED (see below) with its possible complications, but the extracted sperm does need to be used for IVF/ICSI, rather than IUI.

Ejaculatory Duct Dilation

Original treatments designed for EDO included passing long, thin probes into the ejaculatory ducts under the guidance of cystoscopy (a scope through the urethra). Progressively larger probes could be passed in an attempt to dilate any narrowing of the ejaculatory ducts. More recent modifications include a small inflatable balloon on a wire that can be used to attempt to open a blocked ejaculatory duct. These techniques are generally not felt to be as effective as the TURED procedure (see below).

Transurethral Resection of the Ejaculatory Ducts (TURED)

The TURED procedure is done on an outpatient basis under anesthesia and involves advancing a special scope (a resectoscope) down the penis to the level of the ejaculatory ducts (the verumontanum, where the ejaculatory ducts open into the urethra). Portions of the ejaculatory ducts are then carefully resected (cut away) using electrocautery or a laser, thereby relieving the blockage. This procedure is often combined with the injection of colored dye into the seminal vesicles by TRUS prior to the resection. Therefore, when the obstruction has been successfully removed, this colored dye can be seen through the scope flowing through the newly opened ejaculatory ducts.

Success rates for TURED vary widely in different studies. There are many factors that affect whether a TURED procedure will be successful, including the reason for blockage, the location and size of prostatic cysts, the presence of suspected prostatic calcifications or stones, and so on. For example, a big centrally located cyst within the prostate is a sign that TURED may be quite successful for that patient.

In general, for complete EDO, the success rates in returning good numbers of sperm to the ejaculate range from 21 to 75 percent, with the average around 50–60 percent. The rate of natural pregnancy is from 7 to 25 percent.

For incomplete EDO, success rates at significantly improving semen parameters range from 38 to 94 percent, with the average around 70 percent. The rate of natural pregnancy is from 16 to 66 percent. However, 5–10 percent of men with partial EDO also have progressive scar tissue formation and progress to complete azoospermia (no sperm in the ejaculate) following TURED due to recurrent blockage.

EDO is a relatively uncommon problem, so unlike other male fertility procedures (such as varicocele repairs), TURED procedures are not performed very often. Many fellowship-trained infertility experts have performed this procedure only a handful of times during their careers. The TURED procedure also has a significant risk of potentially serious complications. One is watery ejaculate. The ejaculatory ducts usually function like one-way valves that do not allow urine to backflow into them. When portions of the ejaculatory ducts are resected, urine can flow into the ducts and then subsequently come out with the next ejaculation. This problem is generally not reversible.

Another potential complication is recurrent prostatitis or epididymitis. The ejaculatory ducts also help to keep urethral bacteria from entering the genital ducts. After a resection procedure, bacteria can more easily enter, resulting in infections of the prostate and epididymis.

Urinary complications may occur as well. Urine can collect in the resected ejaculatory duct area during urination, and then come out later when the patient is walking around. This can results in leakage of small to moderate amounts of urine into his underpants (post-void dribbling). Another consequence is urinary incontinence. The verumontanum is located right behind the urinary sphincter. If the urinary sphincter is damaged, then this could result in urinary incontinence. This is a rare complication.

Rectal injury is another possible complication. The part of the urethra that passes through the prostate is located above the rectum. Theoretically, if the ejaculatory ducts are resected too deeply, this could result in damage to the rectum, which may need to be repaired surgically. This is a rare complication.

Success rates can be maximized and complications minimized by having a TURED performed by a fertility expert who specializes in this procedure. If you may have EDO and are considering a TURED, I recommend asking any prospective surgeon how many of these procedures he or she has performed. If that surgeon does not perform at least a few of these procedures a year, I suggest you consider finding someone else to do it. Complication rates with the procedure have been shown to be as high as 33 percent in some studies, so you want a specialist who is going to minimize your chances of problems as much as possible. I personally send my prospective TURED patients to Dr. Paul Turek in California, who has performed most of the recent cutting-edge research on the diagnosis and treatment of EDO.

Retrograde Ejaculation

During normal ejaculation, the bladder neck closes so that the ejaculate fluid is pushed forward and out the tip of the penis. However, sometimes the bladder neck does not close completely, thereby allowing semen to flow backward into the bladder during ejaculation. In mild cases, only part of the ejaculate flows backward into the bladder, but in more severe cases all of the semen may be lost into the bladder. Men with retrograde ejaculation may sometimes notice whitish semen in their urine when they urinate after sexual intercourse.

Causes of Retrograde Ejaculation

Alpha-Blockers

Alpha-blockers are medications used for the treatment of benign enlargement of the prostate (benign prostatic hyperplasia, or BPH) as well as hypertension. Alpha-blockers treat BPH by relaxing the prostatic capsule and bladder neck, thereby enlarging the channel through which the urine flows. However, when the bladder neck is relaxed, retrograde ejaculation can result.

Alpha-blockers can also cause decrease emission of sperm (transport of sperm from the vas deferens into the ejaculatory ducts), which can result in complete azoospermia without retrograde ejaculation. In some circumstances, alpha-blockers may even cause complete anejaculation (no antegrade or retrograde flow of ejaculate with orgasm). If alpha-blockers are causing the ejaculatory dysfunction, typically it can be reversed by stopping the medication.

Commonly used alpha-blockers include prazosin (Minipress), doxazosin (Cardura), terazosin (Hytrin), alfuzosin (Uroxatral), tamsulosin (Flomax), and silodosin (Rapaflo). Prazosin, doxazosin, terazosin, and alfuzosin are considered to be non-selective alpha-blockers, meaning that they are less able to affect the types of alpha receptors primarily found within the prostate. These non-selective alpha-blockers tend to have fewer ejaculatory side effects. Prazosin, doxazosin, and terazosin, however, cause higher rates of orthostatic hypotension (a drop in blood pressure on standing) and dizziness because of their effect on alpha receptors within blood vessels.

Selective alpha-blockers (tamsulosin and silodosin) are associated with higher rates of ejaculatory dysfunction. Rates of ejaculatory dysfunction with tamsulosin and silodosin have generally been found to be in the 10–30 percent range. In one study, almost 90 percent of patients taking tamsulosin were found to have decreased ejaculate volumes, as compared to 21 percent of patients taking alfuzosin.

Surgical Treatments for BPH

Any surgical procedures that can open up the urinary channel can also damage the bladder neck, resulting in retrograde ejaculation. Such surgical treatments include:

- Transurethral resection of the prostate (TURP)
- Laser prostate surgery
- Microwave treatment of the prostate
- Transurethral needle ablation of the prostate (TUNA)
- Transurethral incision of the prostate (TUIP)

Urolift is a newer BPH treatment in which sutures are placed transurethrally within the prostate to mechanically open the prostate. Though the data are preliminary, sexual and ejaculatory side effects are reported to be minimal.

Retrograde ejaculation resulting from surgery is typically not reversible. A trial of alpha agonists (see below) could be attempted, but success rates can be expected to be very low.

Diabetic Neuropathy

Advanced diabetes can result in nerve damage throughout the body. This nerve damage can affect the bladder neck, leading to retrograde ejaculation. Good blood sugar control can help prevent retrograde ejaculation in diabetic patients.

Neurologic Disorders

Any neurologic disease affecting the pelvic nerves can result in bladder neck dysfunction and subsequent retrograde ejaculation. Examples of neurologic problems that can lead to retrograde ejaculation include spinal cord injury, spina bifida, and transverse myelitis. In patients with multiple sclerosis (MS), about 50 percent have ejaculatory dysfunction and around 35 percent have orgasmic disorders. These neurologic problems can also lead to complete anejaculation (see below).

Pelvic or Abdominal Surgery

Rectal and aortic surgery are two examples of pelvic procedures that can damage the nerves controlling bladder neck function and result in retrograde ejaculation. Retroperitoneal lymph node dissection (RPLND) for advanced testicular cancer is another surgery that can lead to retrograde ejaculation. These surgeries can also lead to complete anejaculation (see below).

Congenital Abnormalities

Some men are born with anatomic abnormalities of the bladder neck that can lead to retrograde ejaculation later in life—for example, bladder exstrophy.

Diagnosis of Retrograde Ejaculation

The diagnosis of retrograde ejaculation is made with a post-ejaculatory urinalysis (PEU). A PEU is performed by having the man provide a urine sample into a separate cup right after giving a semen analysis specimen. In men with neurologic problems who cannot voluntarily urinate (such as spinal cord injuries), the urine may be collected by urinary catheterization following ejaculation. The lab can then evaluate the urine for the presence of sperm. Small numbers of sperm in the urine are normal, as a few sperm can be left behind in the urethra and picked up by the urine on its way out. However, more than 10–15 sperm per high power field (hpf) on microscopic evaluation is consistent with the presence of retrograde ejaculation.

Treatment of Retrograde Ejaculation

Discontinue Alpha-Blocker Medications

Tamsulosin (Flomax) and silodosin (Rapaflo) seem to be the alpha-blockers that are most likely to cause ejaculatory problems. If the urinary problems are not severe, then stopping the alpha-blocker until pregnancy is achieved is usually the most effective approach. In men with more severe urinary voiding problems, switching to a less selective alpha-blocker, such as alfuzosin (Uroxatral), can often resolve the ejaculatory problems.

Alpha Agonists

Alpha agonists work by increasing the strength of bladder neck closure during ejaculation. In men without bladder neck scarring (for example, those who have not had prior prostate surgery), the success rate in reversing retrograde ejaculation is about 20–30 percent. If alpha agonists are used on a regular basis, their effect on bladder neck function tends to wear off over time. Therefore, intermittent short courses of treatment are recommended.

Examples of alpha agonists include pseudoephedrine (Sudafed), phenylpropanolamine, ephedrine sulfate, and imipramine. Pseudoephedrine is commonly used to treat nasal congestion and sinusitis. It can increase blood pressure modestly, so men with blood pressure problems should check with their primary care physician before they use this medication. Not all formulations sold under the brand name Sudafed contain pseudoephedrine, so check the ingredients to make sure that it does. Pseudoephedrine sales are tightly monitored due to its use in the production of illegal methamphetamine. Some states require a doctor's prescription for Sudafed, but most still require only a photo ID and the signing of a sales log.

Pseudoephedrine can be used in the following manner:

- *Prior to semen analysis (to assess response to treatment).* Take pseudoephedrine 60 mg the night before and one hour prior to ejaculation. (Other published protocols include taking 60 mg four times a day or 120 mg twice a day starting three days prior to the semen analysis.)

- *In conjunction with timed intercourse.* If pseudoephedrine is found to be effective in reversing retrograde ejaculation, then the man can take 60 mg three times a day starting on day 9 of the woman's cycle and continuing the medication for nine days, with planned intercourse every other day during this period (so intercourse on days 9, 11, 13, 15, and 17 of her cycle). Of course, if the woman's cycle is irregular, this schedule may need to be modified.

Sperm Wash with Intrauterine Insemination (IUI)

Sperm can be collected at the time of a semen analysis and PEU and then used with IUI on that day. The urine must be alkalinized prior to specimen collection, as urine is acidic, and this acidity is damaging to sperm. Live birth rates as high as 15–20 percent per cycle have been reported using this type of IUI protocol if no other significant fertility risk factors are present.

Alkalinization of the urine can be achieved by one of the following methods:

- Baking soda (not baking powder): mix 1–2 tablespoons in a glass of water and drink it the night before, and take the same dose one to two hours before ejaculation

- Alka-Seltzer tabs: dissolve 2 tablets in a glass of water and drink it the night before, and take the same dose one to two hours prior to ejaculation

- Sodium bicarbonate tablets or capsules: 650 mg by mouth the night before, and take the same dose one to two hours prior to ejaculation
- Urocit K 10 mg tabs: 2 tabs by mouth the night before, and take the same dose one to two hours prior to ejaculation

Retarded Ejaculation

Retarded ejaculation is the term used to describe the situation when a man has trouble reaching orgasm during sexual intercourse. Potential causes of retarded ejaculation include:

- Hypogonadism (low testosterone levels)
- Medications, especially antidepressants such as SSRIs (Prozac, Paxil, Zoloft)
- Diabetes or neurologic disorders, resulting in poor nerve function and/or sensation in the genital region
- Psychological or relationship issues

When I see a patient with retarded ejaculation, I check a hormone profile to look for low testosterone levels. I also conduct a medication review, looking for drugs that could be contributing to these problems.

Treatment of Retarded Ejaculation

Once a possible cause for the retarded ejaculation has been determined, it may be able to be treated.

- Hypogonadism can be treated if present.
- If SSRIs may be having an impact on ejaculation, considering reducing the dosage, weaning off them, or changing to another type of medication, such as bupropion (Wellbutrin), that may have less of an impact. These types of medication

changes should always be done in close consultation with your primary care physician or psychiatrist.

- Counseling can be an effective means of addressing difficulty achieving orgasm thought to be due to stress, anxiety, or other psychological issues. For guidance on finding a local sex therapist, check the website of American Association of Sexuality Educators, Counselors and Therapists at www.aasect.org.

- Several small studies have shown improvement in ejaculatory and orgasmic function in men taking low-dose tadalafil (Cialis), 2.5 to 5 mg daily. These studies have found improvements in about two-thirds of men taking Cialis, as opposed to only about one-third of men on placebo medications in the studies. See "PDE-5 Inhibitors," above, for more information.

- Cabergoline (Dostinex) is a medication usually used to treat elevated prolactin levels (see "Elevated Prolactin (Hyperprolactinemia)" in Chapter 7). Anecdotally, low-dose cabergoline has been used successfully in the treatment of some men with ejaculatory dysfunction who have normal prolactin levels. The usual dose is 0.5 mg twice a week. If the treatment is successful, most men see a response within the first few months. Potential side effects may include nausea, constipation, dry mouth, gastric irritation, headache, sleep disturbances, vertigo, depression, dyskinesia (involuntary muscle movements), hallucinations, hypotension (low blood pressure), swelling of the hands or feet, arrhythmia (irregular heartbeat), heart palpitations, or angina (chest pain). If you develop any of these side effects, stop the medication and contact your physician. And use cabergoline with caution if you have any of the following medical issues: severe hepatic dysfunction, peptic ulcer disease or a history of GI bleeding, or Raynaud's disease.

Anejaculation

Anejaculation occurs when a man experiences orgasm but no seminal fluid comes out, either antegrade (out the penis) or retrograde (into the bladder). Potential causes of anejaculation include:

- *Alpha-blocker (prostate) medications.* As described in "Retro-grade Ejaculation," above, alpha-blocker medications can cause anejaculation as well as retrograde ejaculation. Higher rates of ejaculatory dysfunction are seen with tamsulosin (Flomax) and silodosin (Rapaflo).

- *Antidepressant medications.* Antidepressants (especially SSRIs, such as Paxil) can cause ejaculatory failure in some men.

- *5-alpha reductase inhibitors (finasteride, dutasteride).* There is some evidence of mildly increased levels of ejaculatory dys-function associated with their use. It is unclear if low-dose finasteride (Propecia) can also cause this problem.

- *Diabetic neuropathy.* Advanced diabetes mellitus can result in nerve damage throughout the body. This nerve damage can cause paralysis of the reproductive smooth muscle, resulting in complete anejaculation. Diabetes can also cause retro-grade ejaculation (see above).

- *Neurologic disorders.* Any neurologic disease impacting the pelvic nerves can result in paralysis of the smooth muscle of the reproductive tract, leading to anejaculation or failure of emission (sperm deposition within the urethra). Examples include spinal cord injury, spina bifida, transverse myelitis, and multiple sclerosis, all of which can also result in retro-grade ejaculation as well (see above).

- *Pelvic or abdominal surgery.* Rectal and aortic surgery are two examples of pelvic procedures that can damage the nerves responsible for controlling smooth muscle contractions of the reproductive tract. Retroperitoneal lymph node dissection (RPLND) for advanced testicular cancer is another surgery that can cause anejaculation. These surgeries can lead to complete retrograde ejaculation as well (see above).
- *Hypogonadism.* Low testosterone levels may cause ejaculatory failure in a small number of men.

Evaluation of patients with anejaculation should include checking a hormone profile as well as a review of their medications.

Treatment of Anejaculation

Once a possible cause for the anejaculation has been determined, it may be able to be treated.

- Treat hypogonadism if it is present.
- Modify medications that could be impacting ejaculation. Stop alpha-blocker medications, or change to a less selective type such as alfuzosin (Uroxatral.) Consider lowering the dosage of any SSRIs, weaning off them, or changing to another type of medication, such as bupropion (Wellbutrin) that may have less of an impact. These types of medication changes should always be done in close consultation with your primary care physician or psychiatrist.
- Alpha agonists are medications work by increasing sympathetic nerve stimulation, resulting in contractions of the seminal vesicles, vas deferens, and prostate. Commonly used alpha agonists include pseudoephedrine, ephedrine sulfate, and imipramine (see "Retrograde Ejaculation," above). In situations involving a failure of emission that is

due to disruption of sympathetic nerve function, these alpha agonists can sometimes reinitiate emission of sperm. Alpha-blockers can also be used effectively in some men with diabetes who have anejaculation. Note, however, that some of these men can still have retrograde ejaculation, so a post-ejaculatory urinalysis (PEU) should always be done (see "Retrograde Ejaculation").

- Several small studies have shown improvement in ejaculatory and orgasmic function in men taking low-dose tadalafil (Cialis), 2.5 to 5 mg daily. Men with more severe cases resulting from issues such as spinal cord injury or previous pelvic surgery will probably not respond to Cialis. However, patients with certain medical problems, such as hypogonadism, may benefit from a trial of low-dose daily Cialis if testosterone replacement by itself is not effective. See "PDE-5 Inhibitors," above, for more information.
- Electroejaculation. See "Spinal Cord Injury," below.
- Sperm extraction combined with IVF/ICSI. See "Management of Obstructive Azoospermia" in Chapter 9.

Congenital Anorgasmia

With congenital anorgasmia, a man has never been able to have an orgasm during his entire life. Most often this is due to psychological issues, which in some men can be related to an overly strict childhood upbringing. Men with congenital anorgasmia often lack a sensual awareness of their bodies. Effective treatment includes sexual therapy with a trained counselor. For guidance on finding a local sex therapist, a potential resource is the website of the American Association of Sexuality Educators, Counselors and Therapists, www.aasect.org. If this is not effective, other treatment options include electroejaculation (see "Spinal Cord Injury," below) combined with IUI, or sperm extraction combined with IVF/ICSI (see "Management of Obstructive Azoospermia" in Chapter 9).

Painful Ejaculation

Pain with ejaculation can have multiple possible causes, including:

- Seminal vesicle inflammation
- Ejaculatory duct obstruction
- Seminal vesicle or prostate stones
- Prostatitis, urethritis, or epididymitis
- Psychological issues

Evaluation of painful ejaculation typically consists of a urinalysis (to look for a bladder infection) and transrectal ultrasound (to look for evidence of problems with the seminal vesicles, prostate, and ejaculatory ducts). Semen analysis testing can be performed to look for pyospermia (see "Elevated White Blood Cells (Pyospermia)," above), which can be a sign of prostatitis or epididymitis.

Specific Medical Problems That Can Affect Ejaculation

Spinal Cord Injury

Injuries to the spinal cord can impact ejaculation in different ways, depending on the level of the injury as well as its severity. In general, about 90 percent of spinal cord injury patients experience some form of ejaculatory dysfunction.

If there are spinal cord lesions at or below T10–L2 (10th thoracic to 2nd lumbar vertebral levels), generally the man can achieve an erection (though without the normal sensation of sexual pleasure), but commonly there is a complete loss of ejaculation.

Men with spinal cord lesions above T10 (10th thoracic vertebral level) generally have an intact nerve reflex arc. These men are often able to get erections, and are also often able to ejaculate.

Men with lesions at about the 6th thoracic vertebral level are prone to autonomic dysreflexia with genital stimulation. This can manifest as bradycardia, sweating, chills, headache, and increased blood pressure, which if not managed properly can lead to stroke, seizures, and death. Autonomic dysreflexia can typically be avoided with pretreatment using oral calcium channel blockers, such as nifedipine 20 mg orally or under the tongue. Men with high (T6 and above) lesions should also have continual blood pressure monitoring during any procedure. Men with very high (cervical level) lesions are at extremely high risk for autonomic dysreflexia, have a higher chance of not responding to nifedipine, and should therefore ideally have all procedures performed under general anesthesia.

Fertility Management of Spinal Cord Injury Patients

Several fertility options are available for men with spinal cord injuries who are not able to ejaculate on their own.

Penile vibratory stimulation (PVS) is considered to be the first-line therapy for men with spinal cord injuries, as it is generally safe, effective, and not too expensive. Devices that have vibratory amplitude of at least 2.5 mm are the most effective. Examples of commercially available PVS devices include Ferticare and Viberect. PVS involves holding a vibrating device against the frenulum (underside) of the penile head for two to three minutes, or until antegrade ejaculation occurs. If no ejaculation has occurred by this time, stimulation is stopped for one to two minutes and then resumed. This can be repeated for up to a total of about ten minutes of stimulation. However, 89 percent of spinal cord injury patients who respond usually do so within the first two minutes of stimulation.

Success rates for PVS depend upon the level of spinal injury. With an injury below T10, there is a 15 percent success rate. PVS is not effective if sacral cord or parasympathetic nerves are affected. Above T10, PVS has an 85 percent success rate.

Several techniques have been developed for use when PVS has not been successful. These include using two vibrators, one on the dorsum and the other on the frenulum of the penis (note that the Viberect device has two vibrating heads), simultaneous abdominal muscle stimulation, and the addition of an oral PDE-5 inhibitor (see the section on these medications earlier in this chapter).

It is always important to watch for autonomic dysreflexia in men with T6 or higher injuries, and to consider pretreatment with oral calcium channel blockers for these men.

Another option is *electroejaculation (EEJ)*. This involves direct stimulation of the penile nerves with an electric probe through the rectum; it can result in ejaculation in most men with spinal cord injuries. EEJ is successful in about 95 percent of cases, although the ejaculation often goes retrograde (into the bladder), so the bladder needs to be catheterized, emptied, and washed out with a buffering solution prior to EEJ, and then the semen must be collected by catheterization following EEJ. As with PVS, It is always important to watch for autonomic dysreflexia in men with T6 or higher injuries and consider pretreatment with oral calcium channel blockers.

Although EEJ is felt to be the treatment of choice in men who are not successful with PVS, several important caveats exist for its use:

- Retrieved sperm can be used in combination with intrauterine inseminations, although success rates can be variable due to the common findings of decreased sperm quality (see below).

- Not all regions of the country have an EEJ machine available for use nearby.

- EEJ is extremely painful in men who have sensation below the waist. In men with no sensation below the waist, this procedure can be performed under local anesthesia. However, in men who have fairly normal sensation below the waist, general anesthesia needs to be used. The cost of doing this procedure under general anesthesia can be prohibitively expensive in some cases.

Sperm extraction is a third option. Sperm can be extracted (typically under local anesthesia) and used for IVF/ICSI (see "Management of Obstructive Azoospermia" in Chapter 9). It is always important to watch for autonomic dysreflexia in men with T6 or higher injuries and consider pretreatment with oral calcium channel blockers.

Erectile Dysfunction and Spinal Cord Injury

Most men with spinal cord injuries (about 85 percent) do regain some level of erectile function by about two years after the injury. However, these erections are not always well-timed or sustained, and only about 10 percent of men with spinal cord injuries are able to successfully ejaculate with sexual intercourse or masturbation. Most men with spinal cord injuries at T10 or above respond well to standard ED treatments, such as PDE-5 inhibitors. These medications can be tried in men with lower (below T10) lesions, but they have a significantly decreased chance of success. Muse intraurethral pellets do not tend to work well in spinal cord injury patients, and this may be due to decreased absorption of this medication in men who perform routine intermittent catheterization. Penile injections and vacuum erection devices can be used effectively, but men with impaired hand function may need assistance.

Sperm Quality in Spinal Cord Injury Patients

If sperm are able to be successfully obtained from ejaculate in men with spinal cord injuries, semen parameters are normal only about 7.5 percent of the time. About 10 percent of these men will be completely azoospermic. There are multiple potential reasons for decreased sperm production and quality in men with spinal cord injuries, including:

- Scrotal hyperthermia from sitting in a wheelchair for extended periods (although this is controversial)
- Infrequent ejaculation
- Problems associated with bladder management
- Accessory gland (seminal vesicle and prostate) dysfunction
- Pyospermia
- Endocrine abnormalities

It is therefore always recommended to check a hormone panel (FSH, testosterone levels, etc.) on spinal cord patients before any fertility-related procedures.

Cumulative pregnancy rates for PVS followed by home intracervical inseminations (ICI) are generally around 20–25 percent. When intrauterine insemination (IUI) is used in conjunction with either EEJ or PVS, per-cycle pregnancy rates are usually around 8–9 percent, although rates as high as 18 percent per cycle have been reported in men with high sperm counts (total motile count over 40 million). Cumulative IUI pregnancy rates are generally around 30–35 percent. Higher pregnancy rates are associated with sperm extractions combined with IVF/ICSI, but these cost more and are more invasive.

Diabetes

Diabetes is one of the most common causes of neurologic abnormalities, and up to 40 percent of diabetic men have some form of ejaculatory dysfunction. The impact of diabetes on ejaculation depends upon the degree of nerve involvement, and can take one of several forms, including:

- Retrograde ejaculation (from incomplete closing of the bladder neck)
- Anejaculation (from paralysis of smooth muscle in the reproductive tract, which is replaced by fibrotic tissue)
- Failure of emission (sperm not deposited into urethra)
- Erectile dysfunction (impacts approximately 35–75 percent of men with type 1 diabetes)
- Calcification of the seminal vesicles (makes them unable to contract and propel sperm into the urethra; EEJ does not work well in these patients)

Management of Diabetes-Related Ejaculatory Problems

Good blood sugar control can help to prevent worsening of ejaculatory problems. The use of alpha agonists (see "Retrograde Ejaculation," above) can convert a failure of emission into retrograde ejaculation, and can also be used to treat retrograde ejaculation itself. In cases of acontractile seminal vesicles, testicular sperm extractions combined with IVF are typically the only option if a couple wants to have a biologically related child.

Post-Surgical Changes

The sympathetic nerves that are responsible for normal ejaculation run alongside the aorta in the deep pelvic and retroperitoneal areas. Surgery in this region (and especially near the aortic bifurcation) can disrupt these nerves and result in problems with ejaculation. Examples of such surgeries include:

- Low colorectal resection (up to 47 percent of these patients have ejaculatory problems)
- Inflammatory bowel disease surgery
- Surgery on the aorta or other great vessels (up to 60 percent risk of ejaculatory problems)
- Retroperitoneal lymph node dissection (less than 5 percent risk of ejaculatory problems if a nerve-sparing approach can be used)
- Transabdominal anterior spinal surgery (up to 20 percent risk of ejaculatory problems)

Damage to the sympathetic nerves in this region can cause retrograde ejaculation, anejaculation, or failure of emission. The severity of symptoms depends upon whether there was total or incomplete disruption of the sympathetic nerve chains.

Management of Surgery-Related Ejaculatory Problems

In rare cases, the use of alpha agonists (see "Retrograde Ejaculation," above) can convert a failure of emission into retrograde ejaculation, and can also be used to treat retrograde ejaculation itself. Electroejaculation can directly stimulate the pelvic nerves to induce ejaculation. Sperm extraction combined with IVF/ICSI is another treatment option (see "Management of Obstructive Azoospermia" in Chapter 9).

Seminal Megavesicles

Enlarged cystic seminal vesicles can sometimes be seen in men with polycystic kidney disease. The cystic changes can render the seminal vesicles unable to contract. These men therefore have semen characteristics consistent with ejaculatory duct obstruction, and evaluation shows enlarged seminal vesicles without evidence of obstruction. As with other problems associated with seminal vesicle dysfunction, brown-colored semen can be found in about 25 to 50 percent of these patients. If a patient with seminal megavesicles is azoospermic, the only effective option for achieving a pregnancy is typically sperm extraction combined with IVF/ICSI.

7

Hormone Problems

Maintaining the correct hormonal environment for optimal sperm production is an important part of managing male factor infertility. This chapter discusses management of any abnormalities found on hormone testing (see "Hormone Testing in Men" in Chapter 4).

A Note on Medications from Other Countries

Medications for the treatment of hormone abnormalities are often expensive and sometimes are not covered by insurance. Prices for individual drugs may vary dramatically between different pharmacies, so call around for pricing if insurance does not cover the medications. This book attempts to identify pharmacies within the United States that offer the least expensive options for hormonal medications. Often medications can be found for greatly discounted prices at pharmacies from other countries, but I don't recommend obtaining medications from other countries, for three reasons:

1. *It is illegal.* The FDA prohibits the purchase of prescription medications from other countries. In the past, the FDA has tended to turn a blind eye to U.S. citizens who travel to Canada to purchase small amounts of medications for personal use, but this activity is still illegal and could come with legal consequences.
2. *Product quality.* In some cases, knockoff medications are produced in second- and third-world countries with little to no control of dosage amounts or production quality. In other circumstances, online vendors

from other countries advertise medications supposedly made by the same companies that supply pharmacies in the United States. However, without official FDA oversight, you are taking their word about the source of the medications they sell.

3. *Confiscation of medications.* When medications are imported, there is the chance that they will catch the eye of a U.S. Customs agent and be kept for further scrutiny. At worst, this could mean permanent loss of the shipment (which has already been paid for), and at best, a several-month delay in receiving your medication.

For these reasons, I always recommend getting your medications from a reputable U.S. pharmacy. Take care when searching on the Internet for affordable medications, as many online pharmacies carrying fertility medications will not reveal on their website what the drugs' country of origin is. When looking into these companies, always ask where the pharmacy is based, and make sure that it is within the United States. Examples of legitimate United States online fertility pharmacies include Walgreens Specialty Pharmacy and Freedom Fertility Pharmacy, among many others.

Management of Low Testosterone

Around 25 percent of men with fertility issues are found to have low testosterone (also called hypogonadism or "low T") on hormone testing. Normal testosterone levels are necessary to provide an optimal environment within the testicles for normal sperm production. Testosterone levels also play a role in libido, erectile function, and ejaculatory function.

There are many different reasons—some reversible, others not—for a man of reproductive age to have low testosterone levels:

- *Aging.* As men get older, they tend to have lower levels of total testosterone. They also have higher levels of SHBG (sex hormone binding globulin), which decreases free and bioavailable testosterone levels.

- *Idiopathic hypogonadism.* In many cases, no specific cause can be found for the low testosterone level, though we can speculate that there is likely some genetic abnormality affecting either the hormonal process that stimulates the testicles to produce testosterone or the actual production of testosterone within the testicles. This is the most common scenario when we find hypogonadism in younger men seeking treatment for infertility issues.

- *Obesity.* This is a known risk factor for hypogonadism, with studies showing that over 50 percent of obese males have low testosterone levels. Weight loss can boost testosterone levels in overweight men.

- *Elevated prolactin levels.* See "Elevated Prolactin (Hyperprolactinemia)" later in this chapter.

- *Excessive alcohol intake.* Reducing alcohol consumption to less than four drinks a week may help.

- *Chronic narcotic use.* Studies have shown that up to 75 percent of men on long-term narcotics have low testosterone levels. Prolonged use of methadone carries an especially elevated risk of hypogonadism. Cessation or significant reductions in narcotic use can help to improve testosterone levels.

- *Varicoceles.* Large varicoceles have been associated with lower levels of testosterone production. Small varicoceles are unlikely to have much impact on T levels. See "Varicoceles" in Chapter 6 for more details.

- *Malnutrition.* Better nutrition may help increase testosterone.

- *Acute illness.* Temporary decreases in testosterone levels may result from an acute illness or from significant trauma to the body.

- *LH deficiency.* Congenital LH production problems are rare and can be treated with LH replacement (HCG injections). Lesions of the pituitary gland (such as a tumor or damage from trauma or radiation) can also result in decreased LH production.

Medications That Can Increase Testosterone Levels

There are two methods by which to increase testosterone levels in men:

- *Giving exogenous androgens.* This involves providing androgens directly in the form of hormone replacement (injections, patches, gels, pellets), anabolic steroids, prohormones, or testosterone boosters. See "Exogenous Androgens" in Chapter 6 for more information.
- *Increased endogenous androgen production.* These medications cause a man's body to produce more testosterone.

A key point in the management of male fertility is that increased endogenous production of testosterone in hypogonadal men can help to improve semen parameters and fertility, while exogenous testosterone administration causes significant drops in sperm counts and fertility. The take-home point: *never give exogenous androgens to a man who is trying to have a child.*

Unfortunately, this seemingly basic concept is not as widely known as it should be within the medical community. I regularly see primary care physicians (and even some urologists) prescribing exogenous androgens to young male patients who are trying to have children. Hypogonadal men who are trying to have children (or who would like to have children in the future) should instead be treated with medications that increase their own endogenous testosterone production.

Increasing Endogenous Testosterone Production

There are three classes of medications that can increase endogenous T production:

- *Selective estrogen receptor modulators (SERMs).* Estrogen normally sends a signal back to the pituitary gland telling it to make less LH and FSH. SERMs block this action of estrogen on the pituitary, and therefore increase the production of LH. This causes the testicles to make more testosterone. Examples of SERMs include:

  - *Clomiphene (Clomid).* This is the most commonly used SERM for male fertility-related hypogonadism. Its use is reviewed in detail later in this chapter.

  - *Tamoxifen (Nolvadex).* Sometimes used for the treatment of male hypogonadism, typically in dosages of 10–15 mg twice a day. Efficacy and side effects are similar to those of clomiphene.

  - *Raloxifene (Evista).* Not generally used in the treatment of male hypogonadism.

  - *Enclomiphene (Androxal).* Currently being investigated for use in hypogonadal men and undergoing FDA review.

- *Aromatase inhibitors.* Aromatase is an enzyme located within the testicles, liver, and fat cells. Its role is to convert some of the body's testosterone into estradiol. Aromatase inhibitors are oral medications that decrease the action of the enzyme aromatase, thereby lowering the levels of estradiol while increasing testosterone levels. (Aromatase inhibitors are also used in the treatment of breast cancer in women due to their estrogen-lowering effects.) Types of aromatase inhibitors include:

  - *Anastrazole (Arimidex).* Anastrazole is the most commonly used aromatase inhibitor for male fertility-related hypogonadism. It is a non-steroidal drug and therefore does not impact adrenal function. Its use is reviewed in detail later in this chapter.

- *Letrozole (Femara).* This medication is commonly used in female infertility treatments but is not generally used for male infertility at this time. Letrozole is also non-steroidal and therefore does not affect adrenal function.

- *Testolactone (Teslac).* Testolactone is used by some urologists in the treatment of male hypogonadism, and it is thought to potentially offer improved benefit for men with Klinefelter's disease (though this remains controversial). The primary downside of testolactone is that it has corticosteroidal activity and can affect adrenal gland function.

- *Exemestane (Aromasin).* Another steroidal aromatase inhibitor. Exemestane is generally not used in the treatment of male hypogonadism at this time.

- *Human chorionic gonadotropin (HCG).* HCG has a mechanism of action similar to that of luteinizing hormone (LH). Like LH, HCG directly stimulates the Leydig cells of the testicles to make more testosterone. HCG is generally considered to be stronger than clomiphene and anastrazole, but it is also more expensive and needs to be given by injection. Its use is discussed in more detail later in this chapter.

Choosing Which Medication to Start With

For the treatment of low testosterone in men who wish to conceive children, clomiphene is usually the first choice due to its ease of use (it comes in pill form) and relatively low cost. If a man's baseline estradiol is relatively high (greater than 45 pg/mL or so), then I consider starting with anastrazole, since clomiphene tends to increase estradiol levels in a significant percentage of men. Occasionally patients are immediately started on the stronger HCG injections without trying oral clomiphene or anastrazole first, such as in men who have been taking long-term exogenous testosterone replacement or anabolic steroids. These men often do not respond well to oral clomiphene or anastrazole, and going straight to HCG is sometimes the best choice.

There is some controversy among fellowship-trained experts regarding the use of medications to treat decreased sperm count in men with low testosterone levels. If FSH levels are normal or high, then some experts feel that increasing testosterone levels does not provide much fertility benefit unless testosterone levels are extremely low. Unfortunately, we don't yet have good clinical data on this. Definitive double-blind studies are difficult to perform, since infertile couples are understandably not often eager to sign up for a trial in which they might wind up in the control group of patients being given a placebo (sugar pill) for a year instead of in the group receiving a medication that could increase their chances of having a baby. Despite the lack of definitive clinical data, I often opt for prescribing medication: we know that sperm are ideally made in a very high-testosterone environment, and if we can bump a man's testosterone level up to roughly normal levels with safe and relatively inexpensive medications (like clomiphene and anastrazole), it makes sense to do so in the interest of optimizing the environment for sperm production.

Response to Therapy

Hormone values tend to respond within one to two weeks of starting a man on therapy. Generally, repeat blood levels are drawn about two weeks after starting any new medication (or after a change of medication dosage) in order to assess the response.

In general, I aim for the following goals for fertility patients:

1. Total testosterone above 300 ng/dL, and ideally near 500–600 ng/dL

2. Free or bioavailable testosterone (only one of these needs to be checked, not all three):

   - Direct (analog) free T: over 15 ng/dL
   - Calculated free T: over 50 ng/dL
   - Bioavailable testosterone: over 156 ng/dL

3. Total estradiol: under 60 pg/mL
4. Total testosterone to estradiol (T/E) ratio: over 10:1

I also look for improvement in the symptoms of low testosterone (which include decreased energy, reduced libido, decreased sexual function, etc.). Some men see improvements in just a few days, while in others it may be three to twelve months before they see maximal improvement.

The spermatogenic cycle (the length of time for a sperm precursor cell to form into a fully mature sperm) is approximately ten weeks long, and so improvement in semen parameters generally occurs over the first one or two spermatogenic cycles (roughly two and a half to five months) after starting medications to enhance endogenous testosterone production. I generally check a semen analysis around ten weeks after starting or adjusting medications, as long as the hormone levels have normalized on this medication regimen, but I remind patients that a repeat semen analysis in another ten weeks may be necessary.

Can Exercise Increase Testosterone Levels?

This is a common question that I get asked, especially regarding strength training or weightlifting. While there may be some evidence that testosterone levels increase slightly with strength training, the evidence is controversial. Furthermore, the increases in blood testosterone levels are minimal and would not be expected to have any significant clinical impact on fertility.

General Protocol for Using Medications That Increase Endogenous Testosterone Production

If a man with fertility problems is diagnosed with low testosterone and started on clomiphene, anastrazole, or HCG, the following is a general protocol that can be used (although individual fertility doctors may have variations of this protocol in terms of timing and tests ordered):

Step 1: Make initial diagnosis of hypogonadism.

Step 2: Start therapy with clomiphene, anastrazole, or HCG.

Step 3: After two weeks, do a blood test (between the hours of 7:00 and 11:00 in the morning). The diagnosis code that can be used for this test is currently 257.2 (E29.1 starting in October 2015). The test should include:

- Total and free testosterone

- Estradiol

- Prolactin (if total testosterone is found to be under 300 ng/dL)

Step 4: Adjust medication as needed (with repeat blood tests two weeks after every medication change) until hormone levels have normalized.

Step 5: Have a semen analysis about ten weeks after hormone levels have normalized.

Modifications to this timeline will sometimes need to be made. An example would be a situation in which time is of the essence, such as when the woman is over forty years old, in which case repeat semen analysis testing may be moved up to an earlier date.

It is important to remember that it takes about ten weeks for a sperm precursor cell to develop into a fully mature sperm, and in order to optimize sperm numbers and quality, the proper environment is needed for this whole period. Taking hormonal medication for just one or two months is not going to have a significant long-term impact on sperm quality. Male hormonal treatments are intended to be taken over the long term, typically until a pregnancy has been established.

Combination Therapy with Clomiphene, Anastrazole, and HCG

Sometimes multiple medications to increase endogenous testosterone production are used in combination. Of course, any time you combine medications you have higher costs, as well as increased potential for side effects.

One combination that typically does not work very well to raise endogenous testosterone production is clomiphene plus HCG. The reason is that clomiphene works by increasing LH secretion from the pituitary, and HCG is already increasing the LH levels in the bloodstream directly. However, clomiphene can raise FSH levels, so if the FSH is inappropriately low in a man receiving HCG, then adding clomiphene to HCG might be of benefit.

A better combination in terms of T production is combining anastrazole with either clomiphene or HCG. Since anastrazole works in a completely different manner than clomiphene or HCG, it can complement their effect on testosterone production while also keeping estradiol levels from getting too high.

For example, let's say a man who has been taking exogenous androgens for low T comes to my office for fertility treatment. After stopping the exogenous androgens, he has a baseline testosterone level of 168 ng/dL with a normal FSH. On clomiphene 50 mg daily his total testosterone increases to only 256 ng/dL, so he changes over to HCG 2,000 IU by injection three times per week. On this regimen, his total testosterone increases to 640 ng/dL with a normal free testosterone, but his estradiol has increased from 30 pg/mL to 85 pg/mL. He therefore decreases his HCG dosage to 1,500 IU three times per week and adds anastrazole 1 mg every other day to lower his elevated estradiol levels. On a repeat test, his lab values are now normalized, showing a total testosterone of 614 ng/dL with a normal free testosterone and estradiol of 48 pg/mL.

If Testosterone Levels Will Not Increase Despite Therapy

Every so often I have a patient who cannot get total testosterone levels above 300 ng/dL despite maximal therapy (HCG 4,000 IU three times a week combined with anastrazole 1 mg daily). In this situation, the Leydig cells that produce testosterone within the testicles are presumably not functioning properly and do not respond to LH stimulation. From a fertility standpoint, one can only maximize the hormonal environment as much as possible with the HCG and anastrazole and then, after the couple is done having children, change to exogenous testosterone replacement therapy. There have been some case reports of men who have developed antibodies against HCG, making it less effective. Antibodies would not be expected to be the problem in men who have little or no remaining testicular tissue because of previous surgical removal or trauma, but they may be suspected in men who have some response to clomiphene but no significant response to HCG. Some experimental treatments have been suggested in an attempt to circumvent the antibody activity (such as plasmapheresis), but no effective standard treatment has been identified. An option would be to try HCG therapy in the form of Ovidrel, since this medication is made through genetic manipulation of bacteria (as opposed to most of the other HCG formulations, in which the HCG is extracted from the urine of pregnant women), and therefore may have a chance of being more effective in the face of antibodies. Ovidrel comes in a single-use pre-filled syringe of 250 µg (essentially equivalent to 5,000 IU of HCG), and this dose can be given as a subcutaneous injection twice a week.

Contraindications to Endogenous Testosterone Therapy

The American Society of Andrology recommends that men with any of the following contraindications should not start testosterone replacement:

- History of prostate cancer
- History of (male) breast cancer
- Untreated sleep apnea (though this is controversial)
- Untreated or severe congestive heart failure

General Health Evaluation for Men on Medications That Increase Testosterone Levels

The American Society of Andrology (ASA) has published guidelines for labs and other evaluations for men who are on testosterone replacement therapy:

- *Prostate-specific antigen (PSA).* PSA is a blood test that serves as a screening tool for prostate cancer. Testosterone makes prostate cancer grow, so men with prostate cancer would not want to increase their testosterone levels. Prostate cancer is rare in young men, and the new American Urologic Association guidelines do not recommend screening for prostate cancer in men less than forty years of age. Men between the ages of forty and fifty-four should be screened only if they have certain risk factors, such as a family history of prostate cancer or are of African American descent.

- *Digital rectal exam.* In this screening test, the doctor places a gloved finger in the rectum to palpate the prostate gland for any nodules or other abnormalities. Along with a PSA test, the digital rectal exam is used by urologists and primary care physicians to screen for prostate cancer.

- *Hematocrit.* This test measures the percentage of red blood cells in the bloodstream. Elevated levels of testosterone can increase the hematocrit in some men, which can increase their risk of developing clotting problems, such as stroke or heart attack. See "Erythrocytosis (Polycythemia)," below.

- *Prostate-related symptom assessment.* Elevated testosterone levels can cause enlargement of the prostate in some men, especially as they get older. An enlarged prostate can block the flow of urine and cause symptoms such as a slow urinary stream and difficulty emptying the bladder. These symptoms are rare in young men but can occur in some circumstances. Assessment for symptoms of urinary obstruction can be performed in older men, or younger men with a history of benign prostatic hyperplasia (BPH, or enlarged prostate) or voiding problems. A simple review of voiding symptoms is fine in most men. Standardized evaluations, such as the AUASS (American Urologic Association Symptom Score), can also be utilized.

- *Osteoporosis prevention/DEXA scanning.* All men with low testosterone levels are at an increased risk for developing osteoporosis, or weakening of the bones, and should receive counseling on osteoporosis prevention (see Appendix E for more details). Though it is not included in the ASA guidelines, I recommend obtaining a DEXA scan (which evaluates bone density) in men with a baseline total testosterone of less than 200 ng/dL.

The ASA guidelines recommend that a baseline evaluation be performed before therapy is started. After treatment has begun, the guidelines recommend additional evaluations after three, six, and twelve months, and then yearly thereafter. However, these guidelines were designed primarily for older men using exogenous testosterone replacement therapy, and these men generally are at much higher risk for problems such as prostate cancer and BPH. What I recommend for the fertility-age population is the following:

- Baseline hematocrit should be performed at the time of repeat blood work after a medication for increased endogenous testosterone replacement has been started (such as clomiphene, anastrazole, or HCG). The hematocrit can then be repeated in about six months. If it is normal at that time, then it is rechecked every six to twelve months while the patient is on the medication.

- PSA screening and digital rectal exam are recommended for the following groups: men over fifty-five, men over forty who have a family history of prostate cancer, and African American men over forty. These screening tests should be performed at the start of therapy, six months later, and then every six to twelve months, by either the urologist or the patient's primary care physician.

- Prostate-related symptom assessments can be done for men who have a history of BPH or urinary voiding problems to see if there are any adverse changes in their symptoms after the start of therapy.

- A baseline DEXA scan should be done for men with a total testosterone of under 200 ng/dL. The scan should be repeated every one to two years thereafter.

(All of these recommendations assume that test results are normal; testing may need to be done more often if abnormal or borderline results are found.)

Erythrocytosis (Polycythemia)

Testosterone stimulates the bone marrow to produce more red blood cells (RBCs). Therefore, when testosterone levels rise, this can sometimes lead to a concentration of red blood cells that is too high, a condition called erythrocytosis or polycythemia. Erythrocytosis can increase the viscosity of the blood, and this thicker blood can lead to an increased risk of clotting complications, such as stroke and heart attack.

In general, medications that increase testosterone levels typically raise the hematocrit by about 3 percent. This rise is usually seen within the first few months of starting therapy or changing dosages; the RBC concentration then stabilizes once a new testosterone level is reached. The risk of having an elevated hematocrit is greatest if total testosterone levels exceed 1,000 ng/dL but can occur at lower testosterone levels as well. If the hematocrit rises above 52 percent, the medications being used to increase testosterone should be modified or discontinued, with a repeat hematocrit blood test done six to eight weeks later. Another option to manage a very elevated hematocrit is therapeutic phlebotomy (blood is drawn and either donated or discarded).

In June 2014 the FDA released a warning that exogenous testosterone therapy may increase the risk of clotting problems irrespective of hematocrit level. It is unclear at this time whether this risk applies to younger men using medications that increase endogenous testosterone production. However, care should be used in men who have known clotting abnormalities, and these men should be cleared by their hematologist before starting use of these medications.

When to Stop Medications for Enhanced Endogenous Testosterone Production

Clomiphene and anastrazole are generally safe to take over the course of several years with proper monitoring. There are some concerns about taking these medications, especially anastrazole, for more than three to five years, as we still have questions about their impact on general medical issues, such as bone health. HCG should be safe to take indefinitely with proper monitoring since it basically just mimics LH, the body's natural pituitary hormone.

All men taking medications to increase their endogenous testosterone production eventually come to a point when they consider stopping them, either because their partner is pregnant or because they have decided to put their fertility efforts on hold. The primary question that needs to be addressed at that time is whether they may want to conceive children again in the future.

Couples Who Want More Children

Couples in which the woman is currently pregnant or who are temporarily putting their fertility efforts on hold but who want to have more children in the future have several options:

- Stop all of their hormonal medications
- Continue their endogenous testosterone therapy
- Switch to exogenous testosterone therapy (hormonal replacement)

For couples who would like to keep their fertility options open, I do *not* recommend switching to exogenous androgen replacement. There is evidence that sperm quality does not always rebound completely when men are on alternating cycles of exogenous and endogenous androgen replacement.

The decision about whether to stop the medications completely or to continue taking clomiphene, anastrazole, or HCG depends on several factors. If the patient had a significantly low total testosterone level (under 250 ng/dL) before therapy began, if a DEXA scan shows evidence of osteoporosis or osteopenia, or if the patient has seen significant improvement in symptoms (such as mood, energy, and sexual function) with increased testosterone levels, then therapy can be continued. However, if total testosterone was only borderline low (over 250 ng/dL) and the man did not notice any change in how he felt while on the medication or felt worse due to bothersome side effects, then he can stop the endogenous testosterone treatment. If the woman is pregnant, I would recommend that the man wait to stop the medication until she has entered the second trimester and everything seems to be going well with the pregnancy. The man can then restart the medications a few months prior to trying for more children in the future.

Couples Who Are Done Having Children

When a couple is 100 percent sure that they are done with their fertility efforts, men with a history of low testosterone should be assessed for the need for ongoing exogenous hormonal replacement therapy. In the United States, exogenous androgens do not come in a safe oral form (due to liver toxicity issues), so some men would prefer to stay on their oral clomiphene or anastrazole rather than switch over to a gel, patch, pellet, or injection. The problem with this approach is that the impact of taking clomiphene and anastrazole on a man's general health over the course of decades is not known. Estradiol levels play an important role in bone health, so the decreased estradiol levels associated with long-term anastrazole use can have a potential negative impact on bone mineral density. Clomiphene does not decrease estradiol levels, but its different impact on estrogen receptors throughout the body could have unknown health consequences when used for decades. To date, studies looking at clomiphene and bone density have shown conflicting results. Further studies are being performed to see if these medications (especially clomiphene) are safe to take for indefinite periods of time, but we will not have the results of these studies for quite a while. On the other hand, exogenous testosterone replacement has been used for decades and is considered to be fairly safe if accompanied by proper periodic monitoring (including hematocrit and PSA). HCG can theoretically be used long-term since it really is just LH, which is a normal pituitary hormone produced by the body. However, the cost of HCG along with the need for injections three times a week has limited the enthusiasm for long-term maintenance usage.

Men who should strongly consider starting ongoing hormonal replacement therapy (if they do not have other intervening health risk factors) are those who have:

- Baseline (pre-treatment) total testosterone of under 200 ng/dL
- History of osteoporosis or osteopenia on DEXA scan
- Significant improvement in symptoms from previous endogenous testosterone therapy (such as increased energy, mood, or sexual function)

For men who do not fall into one of these categories, I generally recommend that they stop their clomiphene, anastrazole, or HCG, wait four weeks, and then get a new baseline total testosterone. I would then consider offering ongoing hormonal therapy to men who have a new baseline total testosterone of less than 250 ng/dL, in order to prevent potential health problems related to low testosterone. I would also consider it in men who developed new low-testosterone-related symptoms during the four weeks they were off the medications (such as negative changes in mood, energy, or sexual function).

Men who switch over to exogenous testosterone replacement should be followed with the same guidelines as for clomiphene, anastrazole, or HCG in terms of periodic hematocrit, testosterone levels, PSA, digital rectal exam, and prostate-related symptom scores (as per the ASA guidelines described earlier).

Management of Elevated Testosterone Levels

Baseline elevated testosterone levels are defined as being over 1,000 ng/dL. Management of elevated testosterone levels depends on the results of LH testing. Possible scenarios include:

- *Elevated testosterone plus normal LH (1.0–8.0 IU/L).* Some men just naturally make high levels of testosterone, and in these men the LH is typically within the normal range. In this situation, I recommend checking the FSH to make sure that it is not suppressed (under 1.0 IU/L). If the LH and FSH are both normal and the patient is not taking any hormonally active medications or supplements, then I would not recommend any hormonal treatment. I would, however, recommend monitoring hematocrit level, since a total testosterone of over 1,000 ng/dL can increase the risk of erythrocytosis (see "Erythrocytosis (Polycythemia)," earlier in this chapter).

- *Elevated testosterone plus low LH (under 1.0 IU/L).* Elevated blood testosterone levels can suppress pituitary production of LH. The most common cause is the use of exogenous androgens in the form of prescription hormone replacement, anabolic steroids, or prohormone/T booster supplements; see "Exogenous Androgens" in Chapter 6. If no exogenous androgens are being used and the LH is still found to be suppressed upon repeat testing, then I would be concerned about another source of excess androgen production, such as an androgen-secreting tumor of the adrenal glands or testicles. Overactivity of the adrenal glands (such as congenital adrenal hyperplasia; see "Glossary of Fertility-Related Medical Problems" in Chapter 6) can also cause elevated testosterone and suppressed LH levels. These men should have an evaluation by an endocrinologist as well as imaging studies of the adrenal glands (MRI or CT scan with contrast) and the testicles (scrotal ultrasound).

- *Elevated testosterone plus high LH (over 8.0 IU/L).* Partial androgen insensitivity syndrome (AIS) is rare, but it can be a cause of elevated testosterone levels and LH. See "Glossary of Fertility-Related Medical Problems" in Chapter 6 for more information on partial AIS.

Management of Elevated Estradiol Levels

Elevated levels of the female hormone estradiol can potentially have a negative impact on sperm production and quality. Elevated estradiol levels can also lead to gynecomastia (enlargement of breast tissue in men).

As described in "Hormone Testing in Men" in Chapter 4, abnormal estradiol levels can come in two forms: an elevated estradiol level (I consider over 59 pg/mL to be elevated, though some people use 50 pg/mL as the cutoff for normal), and an abnormal testosterone-to-estradiol (T/E) ratio of over 10:1.

The clinical impact of elevated estradiol levels on male fertility is controversial, as is the impact of an abnormally low testosterone-to-estradiol ratio. There are currently no definitive clinical data to support either those who think estradiol levels are important or those who do not. I personally try to normalize these levels in order to obtain a fully optimized hormonal environment for sperm production.

There are two ways to decrease estradiol levels: identify and correct reversible causes of increased estradiol levels, or use anastrazole to decrease estradiol production.

Potentially reversible reasons for an elevated estradiol level include obesity (most of the conversion of testosterone to estradiol by the aromatase enzyme occurs in fat cells, and so obese men are at an increased risk for having elevated levels of estradiol), excessive alcohol intake, and use of illicit drugs (such as amphetamines, heroin, or marijuana). Also, certain medications can increase estradiol levels, including:

- Any medication that increases testosterone levels (clomiphene, HCG, T replacement, anabolic steroids, etc.), as elevated blood testosterone levels promote increased conversion by aromatase into estradiol
- H2 blockers, such as cimetidine (Tagamet) or ranitidine (Zantac)
- Benzodiazepines, such as diazepam (Valium)
- Tricyclic antidepressants, such as amitriptyline (Elavil), clomipramine (Anafranil), and others
- Certain cardiovascular medications, including digoxin (Lanoxin), amlodipine (Norvasc), and spironolactone (Aldactone)
- The antifungal ketoconazole (Nizoral)
- The antibiotic metronidazole (Flagyl)
- Finasteride, whether at doses used to treat prostatic enlargement (Proscar) or at the low doses used to prevent hair loss (Propecia)

General health problems that can increase estradiol levels include:

- Hyperthyroidism
- Kidney failure
- Liver failure or cirrhosis
- Malnutrition
- Estrogen-secreting tumors

Tumors of the adrenal glands, testicles, pituitary, or breast can produce large amounts of estradiol. These are very rare, but the possibility must be kept in mind, especially if estradiol levels are very high (over 80 pg/mL) and no other reason can be found, such as a medication that can increase estradiol.

In some men, no cause for an elevated estradiol level can be found. These men probably have a naturally elevated level of aromatase activity as the cause of their increased estradiol levels. This is a presumptive diagnosis, as there is no commercially available way to directly measure aromatase activity.

Assessment of High Estradiol Levels

When estradiol is elevated, I recommend evaluation for potentially reversible causes, including an assessment of medications being taken as well as a review of alcohol and illicit drug use. A more extensive evaluation is indicated in some men where there is some concern about an estradiol-secreting tumor, though these tumors are very rare. Indications for more extensive evaluation include:

- Significantly elevated baseline estradiol levels (over 80 pg/mL)
- Elevated estradiol levels that do not respond to therapy (by, e.g., anastrazole)

- Estradiol levels that continue to progressively increase over time

Men who fit these criteria should have an evaluation by an endocrinologist, as well as undergo the following imaging studies:

- Scrotal ultrasound (looking for testicular tumors)
- MRI or CT scan of the abdomen and pelvis with contrast (looking for adrenal tumors)
- Breast exam
- Pituitary MRI (if pituitary hormone levels are abnormal)
- Mammogram (if scrotal ultrasound and CT scans are normal)

Any imaging findings consistent with a tumor should be immediately evaluated by an appropriate cancer specialist.

Treatment of Elevated Estradiol Levels

Any risk factors that are discovered should be addressed. Such actions could include:

- Weight loss in overweight men
- Decreasing alcohol intake to no more than four drinks per week
- Stopping marijuana use
- Stopping medications that can increase estradiol levels, such as changing from ranitidine (Zantac) to omeprazole (Prilosec)

Anastrazole (Arimidex) provides effective medical treatment of elevated estradiol levels. It works by blocking the action of the aromatase enzyme, thereby decreasing estradiol levels while increasing testosterone levels. This medication is discussed at length later in this chapter. The goal of anastrazole therapy is to normalize estradiol levels to under 59 pg/mL and normalize the testosterone-to-estradiol (T/E) ratio to 10:1 or above. Men taking anastrazole need to be followed with ongoing testing, as described in "Management of Low Testosterone," earlier in this chapter.

Men with a history of an elevated estradiol level should be followed with repeat estradiol levels every six months for a year, and then yearly thereafter while on therapy.

For couples who will want more children in the future, the man can stop taking anastrazole after the woman is pregnant or after they have decided to put their fertility efforts on hold, and then restart the medication three months before beginning to try for subsequent children. Men who are done with their fertility efforts can stop anastrazole therapy and have a new baseline estradiol level checked two to three months later. Mild persistently elevated estradiol levels (60–80 pg/mL) can be followed with estradiol testing every six to twelve months; if the levels remain stable after two to three years, the testing can be discontinued. There is no good evidence that mildly elevated estradiol levels have a negative impact on health or testosterone-related symptoms, but there is some evidence showing that low estradiol levels in men may have a negative impact on mood, sex drive, or sexual function. Men with very high, persistently elevated estradiol levels (over 80 pg/mL) should consult with their endocrinologist for decisions regarding ongoing monitoring and management. There is some emerging evidence that very high estradiol levels might somewhat increase the risk of cardiovascular events, but prolonged anastrazole use can also potentially increase the risk of osteoporosis and bone fracture.

Management of FSH Abnormalities

Low FSH Levels

FSH is the hormonal signal that the pituitary gland uses to tell the spermatogenic cells within the testicles to make sperm. As discussed previously, a normal FSH (1.0–7.0 mIU/mL) is usually consistent with good sperm production, whereas an elevated FSH generally signals a possible testicular problem with sperm production (as the pituitary gland is trying to tell the testicles to make more sperm). However, if the FSH is low (<1.0 mIU/mL), then the testicles may not receive the necessary signal from the pituitary gland, and decreased sperm production can result even if the testicular sperm production "machinery" is normal.

Causes of Low FSH

Possible reasons for low FSH include:

- *Excess androgens.* Elevated androgens can provide negative feedback to the pituitary gland, resulting in decreased FSH secretion by the gland. Exogenous testosterone is the most common cause of low FSH levels seen clinically (see "Exogenous Androgens" in Chapter 6 for more details). Other, much rarer causes include androgen-secreting tumors of the adrenal gland or testicles (see "Management of Elevated Testosterone Levels," earlier in this chapter) or congenital adrenal hyperplasia (see below).

- *Destruction of pituitary cells.* Any process that damages the pituitary gland can impair its ability to produce FSH. One cause of pituitary damage is a tumor. Tumors can arise from the pituitary gland itself or from a structure adjacent to the pituitary gland, and both can destroy normal pituitary cells through tissue compression. The most common pituitary tumor is called a prolactinoma, which is benign (does not

spread to other parts of the body) but can damage the pituitary. Other symptoms that may be associated with tumors in
this area include headache, changes in vision, and deficiencies of thyroid or adrenal hormones. Other causes of
pituitary damage include brain surgery, head radiation,
trauma, stroke, and infiltrative or granulomatous disease.

- *Congenital/genetic problems.* There are some rare but well-
described genetic abnormalities that can result in problems
with pituitary production of FSH. An example of this is
Kallman's syndrome, which can present with a spectrum of
medical findings including anosmia (inability to smell),
midline structural defects (such as cleft palate), and significantly decreased pituitary function; see Chapter 10.

- *Elevated prolactin.* Prolactin levels can exert a negative influence on GnRH release by the hypothalamus, thereby
decreasing FSH production from the pituitary gland. See
"Elevated Prolactin (Hyperprolactinemia)" later in this
chapter.

- *Drugs or medications.* These can include chronic narcotic use,
estrogens or progestins, excessive alcohol intake, or marijuana.

- *Congenital adrenal hyperplasia (CAH).* Excess production of
androgens by the adrenal glands can suppress FSH production and decrease sperm counts and quality. In men with
CAH, testosterone levels are generally elevated and LH levels are low. In a man with high testosterone, low FSH and
LH, and low sperm counts, then elevated levels of 17-OHP,
ACTH, and androstenedione can be indicative of CAH. See
"Glossary of Fertility-Related Medical Problems" in Chapter
6 for more information on CAH.

- *Idiopathic low FSH.* "Idiopathic" means that no discernible reason can be found to explain a clinical problem, such as low FSH production. Presumably the cells in the pituitary that make FSH either did not develop normally or stopped functioning, although the reason is unknown.

A thorough history should be performed to look for any of the above risk factors. If a good reason for FSH suppression is not found (such as exogenous androgen use), then prolactin levels should be tested and a pituitary MRI should be done to make sure there are no structural abnormalities or masses on the pituitary. Other pituitary hormones—LH, TSH, ACTH—should also be assessed to see if the entire pituitary gland is being impacted, or just the cells that secrete FSH. If other pituitary function abnormalities are discovered, consult an endocrinologist. Elevated androgen levels may indicate the presence of congenital adrenal hyperplasia or possibly an androgen-secreting tumor.

Management of Low FSH

Addressing Reversible Causes of FSH Suppression

Discontinue use of all exogenous androgens: testosterone replacement, anabolic steroids, prohormones, T boosters. See "Exogenous Androgens" in Chapter 6 for more details.

If you are taking narcotics for chronic pain, look into alternatives. Consult a pain management specialist to see if you can decrease the dose of prescription narcotics or eliminate them altogether. Also, stop any medications containing estrogens or progestins.

Limit alcohol to no more than four drinks per week, as this may affect FSH levels, and stop all illicit drug use, with professional help if necessary.

Any pituitary tumors that are discovered by imaging should be evaluated by a neurosurgeon, even though many benign prolactinomas can be treated with medicine only and do not require surgery (see "Elevated Prolactin (Hyperprolactinemia)" later in this chapter).

Stimulation of Endogenous FSH Production

When possible, stimulation of a man's own FSH production is usually preferable, since injectable FSH medications are currently quite expensive. When reversible causes of decreased FSH production are found and addressed (such as treating an elevated prolactin level or stopping exogenous androgens), the pituitary gland will often start making FSH again on its own. However, if no reversible causes are found, or if the FSH stays low despite discontinuation of reversible factors, then clomiphene or, less commonly, anastrazole can be used to stimulate the pituitary gland to increase FSH production.

Clomiphene acts upon the estrogen receptors in the pituitary gland to stimulate increased FSH (and LH) production. Anastrazole also has the ability to increase FSH levels indirectly by decreasing estradiol levels (and therefore decreasing the negative feedback that estradiol levels normally have on FSH secretion). Implanted GnRH pumps are available, but they are very expensive and not widely used.

An example would be a man who recently stopped taking anabolic steroids after using them for four years. He is started on HCG injections, and two weeks later his testosterone and estradiol levels are normal but his FSH is still low at 0.1. With time, this man's FSH may rise on its own with just the HCG injections, as he gets further out from stopping his steroid use, but another option would be to add low-dose clomiphene to raise his FSH levels; this may make the sperm return faster.

It's important to note that treatments to stimulate increased endogenous FSH production rely upon an intact pituitary gland. If the pituitary gland has been significantly compromised because of, for example, trauma, surgery, radiation, or congenital developmental abnormalities, then these treatments are less likely to be effective.

Exogenous FSH Replacement

In patients who do not have an intact pituitary gland—for example, those with Kallman's syndrome or radiation damage—or who have failed to respond to clomiphene therapy, then exogenous FSH is often an effective, albeit expensive, treatment.

Exogenous FSH comes in two commercially available forms. Human menopausal gonadotropins (HMG) is FSH that has been extracted from the urine of postmenopausal women. It comes in two types: menotropins (such as Repronex and Menopur), which contain both FSH and HCG, and urofollitropins (such as Bravelle and Fertinex), which contain just purified FSH. The other form is recombinant FSH (rFSH), which contains purified FSH that has been produced in the lab from genetically modified cells. Commercially available forms include Follistim and Gonal-F.

All FSH is given by subcutaneous (SQ) or intramuscular (IM) injection. HMG comes in vials and is drawn up in syringes for use, and Gonal-F is available in this form as well. Follistim and Gonal-F are also available in ready-to-use injectable pens that can be dialed to the selected dose. There have not been any data reliably showing that one form is safer or more effective than the other for male fertility treatment.

The typical starting dose of FSH is 75 IU SQ three times per week, and this dosage is adequate in most men. In some circumstances, FSH dosages can be increased to 150 IU or even 225 IU SQ three times per week, although this can get very expensive. Note that blood FSH levels often do not increase in men taking FSH, as the exogenous hormone does not display much cross-reactivity with most commercial laboratory assays.

After FSH treatment is begun, sperm production restarts in an average of six to nine months; some men respond faster, within three months, while a few others need as much as a few years. Once a pregnancy has been achieved, the FSH injections can be stopped, as there are no other known health benefits of FSH besides fertility.

Injectable FSH may be covered by your insurance company, but if you do not have insurance coverage for your medications, Table 3 of Appendix C lists the prices from some regional and fertility-specific pharmacies.

FSH replacement in men should have minimal side effects, other than mild pain or bleeding at the injection site. If you experience any negative side effects, however, it is best to stop the medication and contact your doctor.

Elevated FSH Levels

As described above, normal FSH levels range between 1.0 and 7.0 mIU/mL. When the brain senses that the testicles are making less sperm than normal, it releases more FSH into the bloodstream to get the testicles to make more sperm. An elevated FSH therefore suggests that the sperm-producing capacity of the testicles is decreased. Elevated FSH is not bad for fertility in and of itself; rather, it is a sign that the brain is responding properly to the low sperm production. There are no medications that can directly lower FSH. The only way to decrease FSH is to improve sperm production (through treatments such as correction of a varicocele, treatment of hypogonadism, etc.).

Normal FSH Levels Despite Decreased Sperm Production

In some circumstances, men with low sperm production are found to have FSH levels in the normal range (1.0–7.0 mIU/mL). Usually the pituitary gland gets signals (from messengers such as inhibin B) that the testicles are making less sperm than they should, and it responds by increasing FSH in the bloodstream to tell the testicles to make more sperm. Sometimes, however, the FSH response from the pituitary gland is blunted, in that it does not produce more FSH in response to decreased testicular sperm production. In these circumstances, increasing FSH levels (through either clomiphene, anastrazole, or exogenous FSH; see above) may stimulate the testicles to produce more sperm.

Management of Thyroid Abnormalities

The thyroid gland is a structure found in the mid-neck region in both men and women. Its hormones regulate body metabolism and energy use. Two primary categories of problems can occur with thyroid function.

In hypothyroidism, the thyroid is underactive. Men with hypothyroidism often experience symptoms of a lowered metabolic rate, including decreased energy and weight gain. There is quite a bit of overlap in potential symptoms of low testosterone and hypothyroidism. Hypothyroidism is typically treated with thyroid replacement, such as levothyroxine (Synthroid). Thyroid-stimulating hormone (TSH) levels are typically high (over 3.0 μIU/mL) in men with hypothyroidism.

In hyperthyroidism, the thyroid is overactive. Symptoms often include weight loss, sweating, and heart palpitations. In hyperthyroidism, the reason for the elevated thyroid hormone levels needs to be investigated. Possible sources include Hashimoto's thyroiditis and tumors of the thyroid gland. Thyroid ablation therapy is typically used to treat hyperthyroidism. TSH levels are typically low (less than 0.4 μIU/mL) in men with hyperthyroidism.

Both hyperthyroidism and hypothyroidism can be detrimental to normal sperm production, but thyroid problems are a rare cause of male infertility. I recommend that thyroid studies be done in male fertility patients only if there are suspicious symptoms present: recent significant weight gain or loss, abnormally low or high energy levels, and sweating or palpitations.

The initial screening test for men with symptoms suggesting thyroid abnormalities is the TSH (thyroid-stimulating hormone) test. TSH is the hormone from the anterior pituitary that stimulates the thyroid gland to produce thyroxine (T4), which is then converted into triiodothyronine (T3). The normal range for TSH is 0.4–3.0 μIU/mL.

If the TSH level is abnormal, you should undergo a full evaluation by an endocrinologist or your primary care physician to make sure that there are no tumors or other medical issues involved. At that time, T3 and T4 levels should be drawn. Normal T3 (triiodo-thyronine) is 80–230 ng/dL. Normal T4 (thyroxine) is 5–14 mcg/dL.

Some male fertility specialists choose to treat thyroid problems themselves, but I usually have an endocrinologist or primary care physician treat these issues. Often they will require lifelong management and monitoring.

Normalization of abnormal thyroid function can improve semen parameters and fertility in men with significant thyroid dysfunction. Mild thyroid abnormalities do not generally result in fertility abnormalities.

Elevated Prolactin (Hyperprolactinemia)

Prolactin is a peptide hormone made by the pituitary gland. It has multiple functions throughout the body, including stimulation of lactation in women. Elevated levels of prolactin (hyperprolactinemia) can inhibit GnRH release from the hypothalamus. Decreased GnRH can disrupt FSH and LH secretion by the pituitary gland, which can result in low testosterone levels and impair sperm production and quality.

Causes of elevated prolactin levels include:

- Medications (the number one cause)
  - Phenothiazines
  - Tricyclic antidepressants
  - CNS-active drugs: antipsychotics, opiates, cocaine, sedative hypnotics, antidepressants
  - Anti-hypertensives: alpha-methyldopa, reserpine, verapamil, labetolol
  - Other medications: cimetidine, ranitidine, anesthetics, anticonvulsants, antihistamines, estrogens, opiate antagonists
- Prolactinoma (functional tumor of the pituitary gland; can cause headaches and changes in vision)
- Macroadenomas (tumors larger than 10 mm)
- Microadenomas (tumors smaller than 10 mm; this is the most common type of pituitary tumor)
- Hypothyroidism
- Stress
- Strenuous exercise
- Nipple stimulation
- Liver disease
- High-protein diet
- Kidney failure (dialysis does not improve prolactin levels, but prolactin levels can normalize with a kidney transplant)
- Growth-hormone-secreting tumors

- Seizures
- Idiopathic (unknown cause; 30 percent of cases resolve on their own without treatment)

Diagnosis of Hyperprolactinemia

The diagnosis of hyperprolactinemia is made by blood testing. A typical hormone profile for a man with clinical hyperprolactinemia is elevated prolactin levels with low LH levels and low testosterone.

Technically, a prolactin level of over 25 mcg/L is defined as hyperprolactinemia. However, mildly elevated levels of prolactin are generally considered not to be clinically significant or cause male fertility problems. Pituitary imaging to check for a pituitary tumor should be considered when prolactin levels are 30 mcg/L or over; most experts order this test when prolactin levels are 50 mcg/L or over, which is what I do as well. An MRI of the pituitary with gadolinium is the imaging test of choice for diagnosing pituitary tumors.

A prolactin level of between 25 and 100 mcg/L may be drug-related, caused by a microadenoma, or the result of pituitary stalk compression by non-prolactin secreting tumor. A prolactin level over 250 mcg/L is usually consistent with prolactinoma, though some medications (such as reserpine or metoclopramide) can increase prolactin levels to over 200 mcg/L. A prolactin level over 500 mcg/L is diagnostic for macroadenoma (mean level 1,415 mcg/L).

Hyperprolactinemia can have no symptoms at all. When symptoms do occur, they may include:

- Symptoms of hypogonadism (decreased energy, libido, erections, decreased body hair, delayed or absent orgasm)
- Galactorrhea (release of fluid from the nipples, which can occur in men)

- Bilateral temporal visual field defects (due to compression of the optic nerve by the pituitary tumor)
- Gynecomastia (breast enlargement in men)

Management of Hyperprolactinemia

When elevations of prolactin are found, any potentially reversible causes should be addressed, including:

- Hypothyroidism (check TSH level; see "Management of Thyroid Abnormalities," above)
- Strenuous exercise
- High-protein meals
- Nipple stimulation
- Medications (see above list)

Mild Elevations of Prolactin

Mild elevations of prolactin generally do not have clinically significant effect on fertility. As described above, pituitary imaging with MRI should be performed for prolactin levels over 50 mcg/L. An assessment of the hormonal impact of elevated prolactin should be undertaken in men with prolactin levels over 50 mcg/L; possible findings including low testosterone, low FSH, or low LH. If the elevated prolactin levels do appear to be having a negative clinical effect, then medical treatment can be initiated (see below).

Tumors of the Pituitary Gland

If any tumors of the pituitary gland are found, see a neurosurgeon for evaluation. Most pituitary tumors are benign and do not require surgical treatment, but a neurosurgeon is best qualified to make that determination.

Management of Drug-Related Elevated Prolactin Levels

Psychoactive medications are a relatively common cause of elevated prolactin levels because they are dopamine antagonists (that is, they block dopamine receptors). Stopping these medications can be difficult in some patients, and therefore one strategy is to bypass the problem by treating the hypogonadism with medications such as clomiphene (see "Management of Low Testosterone," earlier in this chapter). If that does not have the desired effect, then a man can work with his psychiatrist or primary care physician to switch to psychoactive medications with a lower dopamine antagonist potency. If changing medications does not work, one possibility is cautious administration of a dopamine agonist (see below) under close supervision by the primary care physician or psychiatrist. It must be noted, however, that not all patients will normalize their prolactin with this strategy, and the use of the dopamine agonist can exacerbate the patient's underlying medical or psychological problems.

Medical Treatment of Hyperprolactinemia

Dopamine agonists are a class of drugs that inhibit prolactin secretion. These medications can normalize blood prolactin levels and cause tumors to regress, typically over the course of several months. Improvements in semen parameters can often be seen within six months. However, a significant percent of men will continue to have low testosterone levels despite therapy and may require other treatments for hypogonadism, such as clomiphene.

Bromocriptine was the dopamine agonist of choice before cabergoline was available. The typical dosage of bromocriptine is 5–10 mg by mouth daily. Potential side effects include nausea, dizziness, hypertension, and headaches.

However, cabergoline is now the number one choice for the treatment of hyperprolactinemia. More effective than bromocriptine in decreasing prolactin levels and causing tumor regression, it has fewer side effects and higher rates of permanent remission of tumors. It needs to be given only once or twice a week. The initial dose of cabergoline is 0.25 mg twice a week with food. The dosage can be increased by 0.25 mg increments every two weeks, slowly titrating up to 4.5 mg per week if needed, limited by medication side effects (especially nausea, headache, and lightheadedness). Some men may need as much as 11 mg/week to respond. See Table 3 of Appendix C for pricing of cabergoline at several regional and fertility-specific pharmacies.

If no tumor is present, prolactin levels should be checked one month after treatment begins, then every three months for one year, and yearly afterward; once normal prolactin levels have been maintained for six months, discontinue the medication and monitor prolactin levels. However, if prolactin has not normalized by six months after beginning treatment, then consider adding clomiphene or gonadotropins to increase testosterone levels.

If a pituitary tumor is present, prolactin levels should be checked one month after treatment begins, then every three months for one year, and yearly afterward. For a macroadenoma, repeat the imaging tests in three months if the prolactin levels are not improving or if new symptoms arise; if the prolactin levels are improving, imaging should be repeated in six to twelve months. If there are any visual field changes, repeat the imaging immediately, to see if the tumor is impinging on the optic chiasm. For microadenomas, which rarely progress in size, repeat the imaging in twelve months. If two years of treatment have passed with normal prolactin and no visible tumor, the treatment can be tapered off. However, there is a 25–70 percent recurrence rate.

In general, with cabergoline most patients see a normalization of prolactin levels in two months. For patients with tumors, shrinkage occurs in 80–90 percent of cases (compared to 75 percent with bromocriptine). Return of fertility is seen in about 50 percent of men. About 10 percent of microadenomas and 18 percent of macroadenomas do not respond to therapy.

Resistant Prolactinoma

If symptoms are still present, or if there are persistently elevated prolactin levels despite standard medication, then treatment involves increasing the dosage of medications gradually to the maximum tolerable dose. If there is still no response, consult a neurosurgeon about possible ablative therapy.

Risks and Side Effects of Cabergoline

Most side effects of cabergoline are dose-dependent:

- Gastrointestinal: nausea (28 percent), constipation, dry mouth, gastric irritation.
- Central nervous system: headache (26 percent), sleep disturbances, vertigo (15 percent), depression, dyskinesia, hallucinations.
- Cardiovascular: hypotension, peripheral edema, arrhythmia, palpitations, angina. Protracted high dosage use can increase risk of cardiac valve problems (there is no evidence of a significantly increased risk in men receiving standard doses). In men at higher risk for cardiovascular disease, a cardiac consultation should be considered prior to starting therapy with a dopamine agonist.

Dopamine agonists should be used with caution if there is a history of severe liver dysfunction, peptic ulcer disease or GI bleeding, Raynaud's disease, or valvular heart disease.

Ablative Therapy for Pituitary Tumor

As mentioned earlier, a neurosurgical evaluation should be requested for all newly discovered pituitary tumors to make sure that more aggressive therapy is not needed prior to starting medical therapy. However, ablative therapy for prolactin-secreting tumors is generally reserved for patients who have seen no improvement with medical therapy. One of the potential risks of ablative procedures is damage to the other pituitary functions, which can result in pituitary insufficiency. It is therefore important to measure the other pituitary hormones (TSH, FSH, LH, etc.) after ablative treatment.

Types of ablative therapy include surgical resection and radiation therapy. With surgery, 53 percent of patients achieve long-term normalization of prolactin levels without addition of medications. However, 7–50 percent of the tumors recur with time. Risks of surgery include hypopituitarism, cerebrospinal fluid leak, infection, and diabetes insipidus. With radiation therapy, one-third of patients see normalization of their prolactin levels, though it can take years before this happens. Risks with radiation treatment include hypopituitarism, cranial nerve damage, and secondary tumor formation.

Clomiphene

Clomiphene is a selective estrogen receptor modulation (SERM) that competitively binds to estrogen receptors in the hypothalamus and in the pituitary gland, among other places in the body. Estrogen normally has a negative feedback action on the hypothalamus and pituitary gland, so when the actions of estrogen on these structures are blocked, the result is increased secretion of LH and FSH from the pituitary gland. The extra LH secreted then stimulates the Leydig cells in the testicles to make more testosterone. If

FSH levels are inappropriately low, then an increase in FSH secretion can also increase sperm production.

The ability of clomiphene to increase testosterone levels is roughly comparable to that of testosterone gels. Since clomiphene works by increasing LH production by the pituitary gland, if the LH is already elevated (indicating Leydig cell dysfunction), then clomiphene will not be as effective. In men with a baseline LH of over 20 IU/L prior to any medication, clomiphene is not likely to work very well.

Another important consideration is that clomiphene can increase levels of estradiol in some men. The enzyme aromatase converts some of a man's testosterone to estradiol. If clomiphene is started and testosterone levels increase, then more of this T can be converted to estradiol. Therefore, estradiol levels should be monitored in men on testosterone-enhancing therapies.

How Clomiphene Is Used

Clomiphene is taken by mouth. Unlike in women, who typically need to take higher doses of clomiphene on certain days of their cycle, clomiphene in men is taken on a daily (or every other day) basis at lower doses. The typical starting dosage in men is 25 mg a day. Clomiphene comes in 50 mg tablets; some clinicians recommend taking one 50 mg tab every other day, while I typically use 25 mg daily (a pill cutter can be used to halve the 50 mg tablets).

Here is a sample range of dosages:

- 25 mg every third day
- 25 mg every other day
- 25 mg every day (typical starting dosage)
- Alternate 25 mg daily with 50 mg daily
- 50 mg daily
- Alternate 50 mg daily with 75 mg daily

- 75 mg daily (I usually do not go above this dosage, although I have seen clinicians use up to 100 mg daily)

Because clomiphene is much more commonly used in women than in men, I have had pharmacists who are unfamiliar with the treatment of male infertility call the office to question the accuracy of a clomiphene prescription when they see that it is written for a man. I have therefore taken to printing "This is for a male patient" on my clomiphene prescription sheets to decrease the number of phone inquiries from pharmacists.

Clomiphene may be covered by your insurance company, but if you do not have insurance coverage for your medications, Table 2 of Appendix C lists the prices from some regional and fertility-specific pharmacies.

Side Effects

Clomiphene has a bad reputation in terms of side effects, since it can provoke significant mood swings in the women who use it. In men, clomiphene has a good safety profile, and men also do not typically have the same negative mood-related side effects with clomiphene that women do. Most men feel no different while taking clomiphene, and some actually feel better in terms of mood, energy, and libido due to the increased testosterone levels. Adverse side effects do occur in about 5 percent of men taking clomiphene, although these are usually mild. Potential side effects include:

- *Visual disturbances.* Blurred vision, spots in vision, and flashes of light are the most common side effects that I have seen in men taking clomiphene, although they only occur in a small number (less than 2 percent) of them. Generally, the visual side effects resolve within a few weeks of lowering the dosage or stopping the medication. Men with a history of central retinal vein occlusion (CRVO) should consult with their ophthalmologist before starting clomiphene.

- *Gynecomastia (male breast enlargement).* This is the result of elevated estradiol levels, so this side effect should be rare if estradiol levels are followed and kept within the normal range

- *Weight gain.* Typically this is minimal.

- *Hypertension.* Blood pressure should be checked regularly; if it seems to be high, let your doctor know.

- *Cataracts.* An easy, painless exam can check for this.

- *Acne.* This is due to increased skin gland oil production; it usually subsides after a few months of treatment.

- *Dizziness or headache.* More likely at higher doses.

- *Gastrointestinal symptoms.* Stomach upset or nausea have been noted in a few patients.

- *Other symptoms.* Additional side effects that have been seen include insomnia, hair loss, and allergic dermatitis. Aggressive behavior has been noted, though it is a very uncommon side effect.

If you experience any of these negative side effects, it is best to stop the medication and contact your doctor.

There is some concern about using clomiphene in men with congenital vascular abnormalities (such as Klippel-Trenaunay syndrome) due to the potential impact on estrogen receptors within the abnormal vessels. Therefore, anastrazole or HCG may be a better choice in these patients.

Clomiphene and Osteoporosis

The long-term impact of clomiphene on bone density is controversial. Some studies have shown improvements in bone density in hypogonadal men on clomiphene, while others show decreases in bone density while taking this medication. See Appendix E for more information about osteoporosis management.

HCG (Human Chorionic Gonadotropin)

Human chorionic gonadotropin (HCG) has essentially the same hormonal action as luteinizing hormone (LH), the signal from the pituitary gland to tell the testicles to make testosterone.

Commercially, HCG comes in several different formulations. In men, generic HCG, Pregnyl, and Novarel are most commonly used. The three are essentially equivalent in terms of dosing and potency. All three of these medications use HCG extracted from the urine of pregnant women. Other forms of HCG that are less commonly used in men include Ovidrel, Follutein, Profasi, Choragon, and Choropex. Note that blood LH levels often do not increase in men taking HCG, as the exogenous hormone does not display much cross-reactivity with most commercial laboratory assays.

HCG is the strongest medication available to increase endogenous production of testosterone. It is also the most expensive choice and needs to be given by injection, which is why it is typically used only when clomiphene and anastrazole have not been effective. Like clomiphene, HCG can increase estradiol to abnormally high levels in some men.

A common question is whether HCG is more effective than clomiphene or anastrazole. Remember that these medications do not directly improve sperm quality, but rather exert their effect by increasing testosterone production (and, in the case of clomiphene and anastrazole, possibly FSH levels if these are low). Therefore, a man whose testosterone is pushed back up into the normal range by either clomiphene, anastrazole, or HCG should have the same potential clinical benefit to sperm quality. However, HCG is a more powerful medication in the sense of driving increased testosterone production, and therefore it may be effective in men whose testosterone levels have not risen sufficiently with clomiphene or anastrazole. Another difference is that, unlike clomiphene and anastrazole, HCG does not increase FSH production, although this should not matter clinically in men whose FSH is already elevated.

Since HCG works by increasing LH activity, if the LH is already elevated—indicating Leydig cell dysfunction—then HCG will not be as effective. In men with a baseline LH over 20 IU/L, HCG is not likely to work very well.

HCG is not available at most local pharmacies due to a nationwide shortage, and typically needs to be ordered through specialty pharmacies. The shortage is attributed to the popularity of a HCG as a weight-loss supplement, despite controlled studies failing to show any evidence that HCG use actually enhances weight loss. Currently, the FDA deems as fraudulent the marketing of HCG as a weight loss enhancement. The popularity of HCG has also risen through its use by "rejuvenation" clinics for men seeking an improved quality of life and/or sexual function, as well as body builders, who often use HCG between cycles of anabolic steroid use to maintain testicular function.

How HCG Is Used

HCG must be given by injection, either intramuscular (IM) or subcutaneous (SQ). Protocols for injection schedules differ, but most experts recommend three times per week. A typical starting dosage is 2,000 IU three times per week. As with clomiphene and anastrazole, I usually recommend follow-up testing two weeks after starting HCG, or two weeks after any change in dosage or medications. Dosages can then be adjusted depending on the findings of the follow-up blood hormone tests.

HCG dosages can vary widely, from 500 IU to 4,000 IU three times a week. Here is a sample range of dosages:

- 500 IU three times a week
- 1,000 IU three times a week
- 1,500 IU three times a week
- 2,000 IU three times a week (typical starting dosage)
- 2,500 IU three times a week
- 3,000 IU three times a week
- 3,500 IU three times a week
- 4,000 IU three times a week

HCG may be covered by your insurance company, but if you do not have insurance coverage for your medications, Table 2 of Appendix C lists the prices from some regional and fertility-specific pharmacies.

Side Effects

Similar to clomiphene, most men taking HCG do not have any adverse side effects and may even feel better at the higher testosterone levels. However, some uncommon adverse side effects can occur, including:

- Headaches
- Gynecomastia (male breast enlargement; this is rare if estradiol levels are followed and kept in the normal range)
- Weight gain
- Hypertension
- Cataracts
- Acne (due to increased skin gland oil production; usually subsides after a few months of treatment)
- Dizziness
- Restlessness or insomnia
- Tiredness

- Mood changes (depression, irritability)
- Pain at the injection site

If you experience significant negative side effects, it is best to stop the medication and contact your doctor for further guidance.

Anastrazole (Arimidex)

Anastrazole is an aromatase inhibitor. Aromatase is an enzyme located in the testicles, fat cells, and liver that converts part of the testosterone in the bloodstream to estradiol. Anastrazole decreases the action of aromatase, which results in higher testosterone levels and lower estradiol levels. Anastrazole can also raise FSH and LH levels.

A common misconception is that mildly increased estradiol levels play a negative role in men's health, and specifically that it decreases libido and sexual function. Actually, maintaining adequate estradiol appears to play several important roles in maintaining good sexual health, as recent studies have also shown that very low levels of estradiol can lead to an increased risk of low libido and sexual problems in men. The clearest role of estradiol seems to be in maintaining normal bone health (along with testosterone). When estradiol levels are low (under 20 pg/mL) over extended periods of time, there may be an increased risk of developing osteoporosis (see Appendix E). Short-term use of anastrazole (up to a few years) with proper monitoring and prevention strategies is typically fine in most men, but prolonged use may increase the risk of fractures.

High levels of estradiol can potentially decrease sperm production and sperm quality. Another issue is that prolonged elevation of estradiol can also lead to gynecomastia (abnormal breast development in men).

How Anastrazole Is Used

Anastrazole comes in 1 mg tablets. The typical starting dosage in men is 1 mg per day (although some clinicians have begun to use smaller doses, such as 0.25 mg daily; the smaller-dose tablets must be made by specialty compounding pharmacies). I usually recommend follow-up testing two weeks after starting anastrazole, or two weeks after any change in dosage or medications. Dosages can then be adjusted depending on the findings of the follow-up blood hormone tests.

Here is a sample range of dosages:

- 1 mg every third day
- 1 mg every other day
- 1 mg every day (typical starting dosage)

It is generally not recommended to take more than 1 mg daily because of the potential risk of liver toxicity.

Anastrazole may be covered by your insurance company, but if you do not have insurance coverage for your medications, Table 2 of Appendix C lists the prices from some regional and fertility-specific pharmacies.

Side Effects

As with clomiphene, most men taking anastrazole either do not have any adverse side effects at all, and may even feel better because of the higher testosterone level. However, some uncommon adverse side effects can occur, including:

- Increased blood pressure
- Rash
- Paresthesias (sensations of skin tingling, pricking, or burning)
- Malaise

- Peripheral edema

- Glossitis (inflammation or swelling of the tongue)

- Anorexia (lack of appetite)

- Alopecia (hair loss; usually resolves spontaneously when the medication is discontinued)

- Decreased libido

- Erectile dysfunction (2 percent of men)

- Acne (due to increased skin gland oil production; usually subsides after a few months of treatment)

If you experience significant negative side effects, it is best to stop the medication and contact your doctor for further guidance.

8

Developing a Comprehensive Fertility Plan

The goal of the 10 Week Man Plan is to optimize the environment for sperm production as much as possible over a ten-week spermatogenic cycle. When these ten weeks are complete and all of the sperm in the body have been produced in this improved environment, then repeat fertility tests should be performed in order to assess the impact of the interventions. For most couples, this will involve repeat semen analysis testing. However, some couples will be repeating other testing, such as sperm DNA fragmentation testing (see Chapter 11), that had previously been abnormal.

In some circumstances, to save time, some couples may choose to proceed with an intervention from the female side (such as intrauterine insemination or in vitro fertilization) at the end of the ten weeks without repeating formal semen analysis testing beforehand. This approach is fine, and at the time of IUI or IVF cycles the lab generally checks a few basic semen parameters (such as volume, density, and motility), which can provide some degree of feedback to the couple on their male-factor status.

The timeline for repeat testing is sometimes delayed due to certain circumstances. For example, if the dosages of hormonal medications (such as clomiphene) needed to be adjusted multiple times in order to normalize blood hormone levels, then repeat fertility testing can be performed eight to ten weeks after the man made his last medication dosage change.

The majority of men with male factor fertility have problems that are amenable to effective treatment. That is not to say that all men can be restored back to what are considered normal semen parameters. However, the 10 Week Man Plan is designed to quickly optimize a man's fertility potential to the highest degree possible, to increase the choice of fertility treatments for which he and his partner are candidates, as well as increase their chances of conceiving a child.

To sustain any gains in fertility that a man has made on the plan, the changes (in lifestyle, hormones, and so on) must be maintained, or else his fertility parameters will typically revert back to the way that they were before the plan was started. I generally recommend that most interventions from the male side be kept up until the woman is pregnant and through her first trimester.

What if Repeat Fertility Testing Shows No Improvement?

We know that most men with male factor fertility problems have reversible issues, and that addressing these issues can improve fertility potential. However, not all male-factor issues are reversible, and about 25 to 30 percent of men do not show any improvement in their fertility testing results, even after treating all reversible fertility factors that are uncovered during the course of the plan. There are two things to keep in mind in these situations.

First, some men need two spermatogenic cycles to see improvements in their fertility following interventions. It's a good idea to consider repeating fertility testing in another eight to ten weeks to see if more time will result in improvements. Of course, the couple's overall situation needs to be taken into consideration when making this type of decision. If the woman is forty years old and her partner has a total motile count of only 1 million sperm, which hasn't changed after ten weeks of interventions, then maybe they should proceed with IVF/ICSI if possible, since her age makes waiting an additional two and a half months potentially undesirable. In such circumstances, good communication between the couple and their fertility physicians is especially important.

Second, some men have improved fertility potential even though there is no detectable change in their basic semen parameters. We know that the semen parameters of density, motility, and morphology are not the whole story of male fertility potential. Sperm DNA fragmentation testing is just one of many other male fertility tests that will eventually be developed and refined to provide further fertility potential information beyond knowing just how many sperm are present, how well they swim, and how many have normal shapes. The interventions described in this book may improve a man's fertility even if his semen parameters do not change appreciably, so I urge men in this situation to continue to follow the plan's guidelines.

Developing a Global Plan

As discussed at the beginning of this book, successful fertility efforts always need to take into account both the male and female factors that are present. The 10 Week Man Plan focuses on improving male fertility parameters to the fullest extent possible. Once this has been accomplished, the next step is to assess where things stand for both members of the couple and to develop a plan that is going to achieve their fertility goals as effectively as possible.

There is no one strategy that is applicable to all couples; each plan must be based upon their individual situations. Some couples are just starting the fertility treatment process, while others have already undergone multiple interventions (like IUI and IVF) without success. Others are dealing with abnormal sperm DNA fragmentation levels or recurrent unexplained pregnancy loss. Depending on the results of repeat fertility testing after the initial ten weeks, individual couples will have to decide how to proceed. Perhaps they will try another cycle of IVF now that the DNA fragmentation levels have normalized, or they will go ahead with another cycle of IUI since the total motile count has improved by 50 percent.

For couples that are just starting down the fertility treatment path, deciding on the next step can be an intimidating process. As discussed in Chapter 5, women should undergo a basic female fertility evaluation by an ob-gyn or a specialist in female fertility, and this can often be accomplished while the man is going through the 10 Week Man Plan. Taking into account both the female and male fertility issues that are present can help to determine this next course of action. Open, honest communication between the couple and their respective medical care providers is very important to establishing an effective and efficient global fertility plan.

Typically, once the male parameters have been optimized, the focus will shift to interventions from the female side that can enhance the chances of successful interventions. Some couples in whom significant improvements in sperm counts have been seen with the 10 Week Man Plan may simply decide to try natural timed intercourse for several more months, and this is a reasonable plan, especially if the woman is young. However, most couples who are using the plan have been trying to conceive for at least 6 to 12 months, so pursuing interventions from the female side may increase the chances of reproductive success. These interventions include:

- Medications for the woman, such as clomiphene, tamoxifen, letrozole, or anastrazole
- Intrauterine insemination (IUI)

- In vitro fertilization (IVF)
- Intracytoplasmic sperm injection (ICSI)

Appendix D reviews these female-side treatments in more detail.

Choosing the Right Female Treatments for a Couple

From the woman's side, many different factors can play a role in determining which types of treatments she is a candidate for. Examples of these factors include whether the woman is ovulating normally, if her fallopian tubes are blocked, how good her ovulatory reserve is, and whether she has any uterine or cervical abnormalities.

From the male side of things, the total motile count (TMC) is usually the most predictive factor as to what types of treatments the couple is a candidate for (see "Semen Analysis Results" in Chapter 3 for more information on TMC). One of the goals of the 10 Week Man Plan is to increase TMC as much as possible, so as to improve the range of treatment options available to a couple. The following are general guidelines for the number of sperm that make a couple eligible for the different treatment options available from the female side:

Female fertility treatment	Minimum total motile count (TMC) to be considered a candidate	Ideal TMC for this type of procedure
Natural intercourse combined with hormones (e.g., clomiphene, letrozole)	10 million	20 million or more
Intrauterine insemination	5 million pre-wash 1 million post-wash	20 million or more pre-wash 5 million or more post-wash
Standard IVF	100,000 sperm/cc (regular density)	1 million/cc or more
IVF/ICSI	5–20 live sperm	100,000/cc or more

These are only general recommendations, and the exact clinical circumstances should always be used to make the final decisions on what course of action to pursue. In general, for couples with decent semen parameters that make them candidates for any of the above listed female fertility treatments, a step-wise progression is often recommended. If natural intercourse has not been successful after twelve months, then a trial of timed intercourse combined with medications (such as clomiphene or letrozole) is tried. If this has not been successful after three or four cycles, then the couple moves on to intrauterine insemination. If IUI does not produce results after three or four cycles, then the couple generally moves on to IVF.

Many factors can modify the course of treatment, however. If the woman is older, then moving more quickly to a more aggressive form of treatment (such as IUI or IVF) may be indicated. Also, some couples who have been trying for a long time may not wish to wait any longer, and prefer to move straight to a more aggressive intervention. For couples in which the man's sperm count is borderline to be considered to be a candidate for an intervention, the couple may also choose to modify their approach. For example, a man with a pre-wash TMC of 5 million sperm may choose to try only one or two cycles of IUI (instead of the standard three or four cycles) before moving on to IVF if no pregnancy has been established.

The formulation of a fertility management plan that is specific for each particular couple and takes into consideration both the male and female factors present is extremely important to optimizing the chances of establishing a pregnancy. Excellent communication and coordination of care between the man's and woman's fertility specialists is vital to successfully forming a treatment plan for the couple and maximizing their chances of success.

9

Virtual Azoospermia and Azoospermia

Some men who are having trouble conceiving are found to have extremely low sperm counts. Virtual azoospermia is defined as having fewer than 100,000 sperm/cc in the ejaculate, while azoospermia means having absolutely no sperm in the ejaculate whatsoever.

Virtual Azoospermia

Virtual azoospermia, which denotes a very low sperm count, can be described in several different ways. The most common way is perhaps the estimated number of sperm per cubic centimeter—for example, 100,000 sperm per cc (also written as 0.1×10^6/cc). You may also see this written as number of sperm per high-power field (HPF). For example, with an uncentrifuged specimen, you might see "3 sperm seen on entire slide" or "3 sperm seen on Makler" (the Makler chamber is the counting chamber used to measure the sperm count and motility in one drop of semen). When a centrifuged (that is, concentrated) specimen is examined, you might see a report like "8 sperm seen in centrifuged specimen, 2 of which were motile"—this generally represents all of the sperm in the entire ejaculate, as opposed to just the amount of sperm in one drop of the ejaculate. Of course, only 8 sperm seen in a concentrated specimen is going to represent a more severe problem than 8 sperm seen in only one drop of the semen.

Patients with virtual azoospermia can sometimes have such low sperm counts that not enough sperm are present to proceed with IVF/ICSI. The lab that is planning on doing the IVF should have its own technicians evaluate the semen and decide whether they think there is enough sperm to inject all of the eggs they anticipate retrieving. This decision is made in consultation with the IVF doctor, who can often roughly estimate the number of expected eggs based upon the woman's age and ovulatory reserve.

Freezing of Sperm for Men with Virtual Azoospermia

Freezing (cryopreservation) of sperm is always a good idea in men with sperm counts of under 1 or 2 million sperm/cc. In this case, if enough sperm are not present on the day of IVF egg retrieval, then the lab can thaw out the backup frozen sperm to use. Another option would be to freeze (vitrify) the eggs (see "Management of Non-Obstructive Azoospermia," later in this chapter).

The problem with sperm cryopreservation, however, is that approximately 50–75 percent of sperm do not survive the freeze-and-thaw process. (In better-quality specimens, higher percentages of sperm typically survive being frozen.) Freezing good numbers of sperm is generally not a problem in men with higher sperm counts. However, sperm from men with virtual azoospermia typically do not freeze well, and with such men the thawed semen specimen may not yield any sperm that are alive and usable for IVF. The IVF lab needs to decide, based on the sperm density and quality of a particular fresh specimen, whether they think they will be able to retrieve sperm after the freeze-thaw process for that specimen. It's important to realize that relative sperm quality can change from sample to sample in the same person, since every man's semen parameters fluctuate from week to week, so providing several specimens for preservation may be necessary for the lab to make this determination. Some labs freeze a smaller test sample, which they can then thaw out to check the post-thaw quality of the specimen.

Management of Virtual Azoospermia

The primary goal of managing virtual azoospermia is to address any reversible factors that can potentially increase sperm counts and quality. Examples of these reversible factors include hormone abnormalities, varicoceles, lifestyle factors (such as use of hot tubs or saunas, smoking, and so on), and medications that might be detrimental to sperm production.

In general, if men start off in the virtual azoospermia range, success typically means getting sperm counts up to a point where there are plenty of sperm for IVF/ICSI. There are exceptions in which sperm counts may rise to the point of potential conception using IUI or even natural intercourse (examples would include men who had previously been on exogenous androgens, or perhaps who have had a very large varicocele treated). However, most men with only a few sperm to start will not be able to raise their counts up to a point at which IUI is possible.

If sperm counts improve to the point at which the IVF doctor and lab feel comfortable that enough sperm will be available to inject most or all of the eggs, then proceeding with IVF/ICSI is the next step. A double collection of sperm (two ejaculated specimens) on the day of egg retrieval can sometimes be useful in finding more fresh sperm. Ideally, the man would also have some backup frozen sperm in case his ejaculated sperm counts were lower on the day of egg retrieval. If no frozen backup specimens are available because counts were too low (or if the frozen specimens are of questionable quality), then the option of donor sperm as a backup should be considered (see Appendix F), as should freezing any uninjected eggs (see "Management of Non-Obstructive Azoospermia," later in this chapter).

If, after all reversible factors have been addressed, sperm counts are still considered too low for IVF/ICSI, then a fresh testicular biopsy can be considered. By going straight to the source of sperm production, enough live sperm can be found to inject all of the retrieved eggs approximately 50 percent of the time in men with virtual azoospermia (see "Management of Obstructive Azoo-spermia," later in this chapter for more information on sperm extraction techniques). Ideally, this sperm retrieval would be timed with the day of the woman's egg retrieval. The coordination of these two procedures can be challenging from a logistical stand-point, since the timing of the exact date when the woman's eggs will be ready for retrieval is not known until a few days prior. Donor sperm backup or preparations for freezing eggs should be considered in these circumstances, in case enough sperm are not found in the testicular tissue.

Azoospermia

There are three possible reasons for azoospermia, or a complete lack of sperm in the ejaculate when tested. These include sperm production problems (also called non-obstructive azoospermia, or NOA), blockage problems (also called obstructive azoospermia, or OA), and ejaculatory or sperm transport problems.

Figuring out which of the above reasons is causing the azoo-spermia involves a detailed evaluation, including blood hormone testing, a physical exam, and a review of the man's medical history and any medications or supplements he is taking. However, two factors—FSH and testicular volume—are usually fairly accurate at narrowing down which of the above problems is present.

FSH is the hormone from the brain that tells the testicles to make sperm (see "Hormone Testing in Men" in Chapter 4). If the

FSH is normal (1–7 IU/L), then it is more than 90 percent accurate in predicting that sperm production is normal. A high FSH is generally consistent with abnormal sperm production, because when the brain receives information that the testicles are making less sperm than normal, it secretes more FSH to signal the testicles to make more sperm. However, sometimes a man can have a severe sperm production problem but still have a normal FSH and testicular size. In this scenario, called maturation arrest, the testicles make large numbers of sperm "parts" but are not putting them together into normal functioning sperm (see "Maturation Arrest," below).

Normal testicular size is considered to be 20cm³ or more (see "Fertility-Related Physical Exam" in Chapter 4). Most of the volume of the testicles is made up of the cells that produce sperm. Therefore, if the testicles are not making many sperm, then the spermatogenic cells are usually atrophic (small) or nonexistent. The size of the testicles in men with low sperm production is therefore usually smaller than normal (a condition called atrophy). But as with FSH, men with maturation arrest can have testicles that are busy making sperm parts (though not complete sperm) and therefore may be of normal size.

Low FSH and Azoospermia

When the FSH is low (under 1.0 mIU/mL), then we have to consider that something might be suppressing pituitary function. In this scenario, the brain is not sending the signal (FSH) to the testicles to tell it to make sperm. Potential reasons for this include:

- Exogenous androgen use (see "Exogenous Androgens" in Chapter 6)
- Pituitary insufficiency as a result of illness, surgery, or trauma (see "Glossary of Fertility-Related Medical Problems" in Chapter 6)

- Congenital absence of FSH production, such as with Kall-man's syndrome (see Chapter 10)

- Congenital adrenal hyperplasia (see "Glossary of Fertility-Related Medical Problems" in Chapter 6)

- Androgen-secreting tumor (for example, adrenal or testicular tumor)

See "Management of FSH Abnormalities" in Chapter 7 for further information on diagnosing and treating low FSH levels.

Normal FSH and Azoospermia

A normal FSH blood test (1.0–7.0 MIU/ml) typically indicates normal sperm production. However, this test is not 100 percent accurate, as the FSH can be falsely elevated in conditions such as maturation arrest. Potential reasons for azoospermia in men with a normal FSH include:

- Blockage problem (obstructive azoospermia)

- Ejaculatory problem

- Genital duct sperm transport problem

- Maturation arrest (see below)

The following steps can be taken to help figure the cause of azoospermia in men with a normal FSH:

1. Review the medical history for potential causes of sperm blockage.

   - *Previous scrotal/inguinal surgery.* This includes inguinal hernia repair, hydrocele repair, or undescended testicle repair. In adults, the risk of injury to the vas deferens during the repair of an inguinal hernia is 0.8–2 percent, while the risk of damage to the testicular blood supply is 1–5 percent. For children, the risk of injury to the vas during inguinal hernia repair is higher, at 10–27 percent, with the risk of damage to the testicular blood supply at 2–5 percent. The risk of injury to the epididymis during a hydrocelectomy is 5.5 percent, while risk of epididymal injury during spermatocelectomy is 17 percent.

- *Scrotal trauma.* Every man has had some incidents of scrotal trauma, and severe trauma can result in damage to the testicle and genital duct system. Most scrotal trauma (kicks to the area, bike accidents, etc.) do not cause significant damage. In general, if you did not have to go to the emergency room for the trauma, then it likely was not significant enough to damage the scrotal contents.

- *Previous abdominal/pelvic surgery or trauma.* The vas deferens runs through the pelvis and deep abdominal area in its route from the testicles to the urethra. Abdominal or pelvic surgery or significant trauma can potentially disrupt the vas deferens in this area.

- *Gonadal duct infections.* Most infections that affect the gonadal duct, such as chlamydia and gonorrhea, do not cause obstruction, but some infections can be associated with intense inflammation in the ducts, which can lead to scarring and blockage. Some reports have found that the HPV virus (which causes genital warts) can be associated with ductal scarring, but the vast majority of men with HPV do not have subsequent blockage issues.

2. Do a physical exam.

- *Vas deferens.* Can a normal vas deferens be palpated on each side?

- *Epididymis.* Is the epididymis engorged, enlarged, or absent?

- *Testicles.* Is the testicular size normal?

3. Review all medications and supplements being taken. Some medications, especially SSRI antidepressants, can cause decreased ductal transport of sperm. Alpha blockers (used to treat prostate enlargement and hypertension) can also cause decreased ductal transport as sperm as well as retrograde ejaculation.

4. Review the sexual history.

   - *Erections and orgasm.* Does the patient have any problems with getting or keeping an erection, or with reaching orgasm?

   - *Ejaculation.* Does semen come out of the penis when he ejaculates?

   - *Semen.* Any recent changes in the volume or quality of the semen?

5. Review the medical history.

   - *Neurologic problems.* Conditions such as multiple sclerosis, spinal cord injury, and so on can decrease ductal transport of sperm as well as affect ejaculation.

   - *Diabetes.* Diabetes-related neurologic changes can affect ejaculation and ductal transport of sperm. Diabetes can also lead to calcification of the seminal vesicles, which can decrease their ability to contract during ejaculation.

   - *Polycystic kidney disease.* This can result in cystic changes in the seminal vesicles that prevent effective contraction with ejaculation.

6. Check ejaculate volume (see "Reversible Semen Parameter Factors" in Chapter 6). The normal amount of semen fluid passed during ejaculation is 1.0 cc or more. A low ejaculate volume (under 1.0 cc) can be due to incomplete collection of

the specimen), blockage, or retrograde ejaculation. Low testosterone levels can also cause decreases in ejaculate volume as well.

7. Evaluate semen fructose and pH (see "Reversible Semen Parameter Factors" in Chapter 6). The seminal vesicles make most of the ejaculate volume. Seminal vesicle fluid is alkaline in pH and contains fructose. By contrast, the prostatic fluid has an acidic pH and does not contain fructose. Since the seminal vesicles produce the majority of the fluid, the overall pH of normal semen is alkaline (pH between 7.2 and 7.5). The ejaculatory ducts join the vas deferens to the ducts draining the seminal vesicles, whereupon the semen enters the prostatic urethra at the verumontanum along with the prostatic fluid. If the ejaculatory ducts are completely blocked, then the fluid from the testicles and seminal vesicles is blocked, and only the prostatic fluid comes out with ejaculation. If the semen is acidic and has no fructose, then fluid from the seminal vesicles and testicles is not making it into the ejaculate.

8. Do a post-ejaculatory urinalysis (PEU). If there is a suspicion of ejaculatory problems (such as low ejaculate volume), then a PEU should be performed to look for the presence of retrograde ejaculation. See "Ejaculatory Problems" in Chapter 6.

Common Clinical Findings in Azoospermic Men with Normal FSH and Testicular Volume

Blockage Problems (Obstructive Azoospermia)

Men with obstructive azoospermia often have a history of trauma, surgery, or infection. On physical exam, the doctor may find no palpable vas deferens on one or both sides (consistent with possible

CBAVD; see Chapter 10). A dilated epididymis on each side can be consistent with congenital epididymal obstruction (blockage of epididymal tubules on each side that has been present since birth). A semen analysis that shows a normal semen volume (1.0 cc or more), normal pH (7.2–7.5), and the presence of fructose indicates that the blockage does not involve the ejaculatory ducts.

On the other hand, if the ejaculatory ducts are blocked, the semen analysis is likely to show low ejaculate volume (under 1.0 cc), a low pH (under 7.2), and the absence of fructose. This can be due to ejaculatory duct obstruction (see "Ejaculatory Problems" in Chapter 6) or congenital bilateral absence of the vas deferens (see Chapter 10).

Ejaculatory Problems

In men with azoospermia related to ejaculatory problems, typically the semen analysis will show a low semen volume (under 1.0cc) with a normal pH (7.2–7.5) and the presence of fructose. Problems with ejaculation may be seen in men with a history of prior pelvic surgery, men with a neurologic disorder, and men who take medications (such as SSRI antidepressants or alpha blockers) that can disrupt normal ejaculation.

Sometimes men with retrograde ejaculation have a history of milky-colored urine when they void following ejaculation.

Genital Duct Sperm Transport Problems

Problems with transport of sperm in the genital ducts may be indicated by a semen analysis that shows a normal semen volume (1.0 cc or more), normal pH (7.2–7.5), and the presence of fructose. Sperm transport problems resulting in azoospermia may occur in men who have a history of pelvic surgery, who have a neurologic disorder, who use medication that can disrupt normal ejaculation (such as SSRI antidepressants or alpha blockers), or who have diabetes or polycystic kidney disease.

Maturation Arrest

If an azoospermic man's semen analysis shows normal semen volume (over 1.0 cc), normal pH (7.2–7.5), and the presence of fructose, maturation arrest may be suspected if there is no history of surgery or trauma that could cause sperm blockage.

Obstructive Azoospermia vs. Maturation Arrest

Ejaculatory and ductal sperm transport problems are usually fairly straightforward to identify. Men with ejaculatory problems usually have either a low ejaculate volume or a clearly evident problem with reaching orgasm. Genital duct transport issues are usually accompanied by a history of neurologic problems or the use of medications such as alpha blockers or anti-depressants, with the sperm returning after the medications are discontinued. Some causes of obstruction are also fairly easy to diagnose, such as men who do not have a palpable vas on each side, or who had a complicated bilateral hernia repair as a child.

Sometimes, however, the cause of the azoospermia is less clear. An example would be an azoospermic man who has not conceived children in the past and who has a normal FSH, normal testicular size, a normal palpable vas deferens on each side, normal semen volume and pH, fructose in the semen, and no reason in his history for possible blockage or sperm transport problems. Is this a congenital blockage deep in the pelvis involving the vas deferens on both sides, or is this actually maturation arrest with severe sperm production problems (see "Maturation Arrest" later in this chapter)? Sometimes the only way to find out is with a testicular biopsy, in which a small number of testicular tubules are removed and evaluated for the presence of sperm. If no sperm are found, then the condition should be managed as non-obstructive azoo-spermia (see "Management of Non-Obstructive Azoospermia," later in this chapter). If sperm are found, then this is consistent with a blockage at an unknown location. Any retrieved sperm should be frozen at the time of the biopsy so that they can be used for IVF/ICSI in the future. Surgical exploration can be considered to try to locate a potentially reconstructable area of obstruction, although if the area of obstruction is deep within the pelvis, then it is not typically considered to be reconstructable.

Indirect anti-sperm antibody testing can sometimes be helpful in distinguishing azoospermia caused by blockage from azoo-spermia caused by maturation arrest (see "Clumping of Sperm and Anti-Sperm Antibodies" in Chapter 6). About 70 percent of men with acquired obstructive azoospermia will be positive for anti-sperm antibodies on indirect ASA testing of the blood, whereas men with nonobstructive azoospermia typically should not be positive for anti-sperm antibodies. Note, however, that men with a congenital blockage (one that has existed since birth) typically do not have elevated levels of anti-sperm antibodies. This information may help to guide treatment options, though a definitive diagnosis cannot be made without testicular biopsy, as described above.

Treating Azoospermia

Obstructions resulting in azoospermia are generally managed in one of two ways: surgical reconstruction or sperm extraction combined with IVF/ICSI. These topics are covered in "Management of Obstructive Azoospermia" later in this chapter.

When the azoospermia is a result of issues with ejaculation, see "Ejaculatory Problems" in Chapter 6.

If sperm transport problems are suspected, the first solution is to try to identify any reversible causes, such as the use of SSRI antidepressants or the use of alpha blockers, especially tamsulosin and silodosin. (Any medication changes should be done only under the close supervision of a medical professional.) If this is not effective, then sperm extraction combined with IVF/ICSI is an option.

Management of Maturation Arrest

See "Management of Non-Obstructive Azoospermia" later in this chapter.

High FSH and Azoospermia

When a man has azoospermia and an elevated FSH (especially if it is over 10–15 MIU/ml), then most likely a severe sperm production problem is the cause of the azoospermia. This is typically referred to as non-obstructive azoospermia (NOA). An important point to remember is that this does not necessarily mean that no sperm are being made, but only that none were seen by the lab in that specific semen sample. Sperm production must reach a certain threshold level for sperm to start "spilling over" into the ejaculate. Sometimes men who are azoospermic on one sample have small amounts of sperm in subsequent samples. Studies have shown that men who have had two consecutive semen analyses showing complete azoospermia (and who have no other reversible causes) have about a 20 percent chance of finding small amounts of sperm on a third analysis, a 10 percent chance on a fourth analysis, and then a less than 1 percent chance on subsequent analyses. For azoospermic men in whom I suspect a production problem, I usually check at least three semen specimens, ideally all at least ten weeks apart.

There can be a variety of causes for non-obstructive azoospermia (NOA):

- *Testicular damage.* Severe trauma to the testicles can sometimes damage them to the point where sperm production stops. With time, some production may return, but in some cases the damage has been so severe that sperm production never returns.

- *Infection.* Bacterial and viral testicular infections can disrupt normal sperm production. Production typically returns with time in most men, but in some circumstances (such as orchitis resulting from mumps) the damage can be permanent. Also, systemic body infections (that is, infections of the body that do not directly involve the testicles themselves—for example, flu with a high fever) can place enough stress on the body to temporarily cause sperm production to decrease or stop altogether. Sperm production in these men typically recovers with time, but it can take three to six months, or even longer in some circumstances.

- *Less than optimal environment for sperm production.* Of course, a poor environment for sperm production might also be the cause of NOA. One of the primary goals of male infertility management is to try to optimize the environment for sperm production as much as possible. There are a variety of negative environmental factors that can decrease sperm production in some men, including the use of hot tubs or saunas, taking very hot showers, using a laptop computer directly on the lap, and so on. By themselves, these environmental factors typically do not result in complete azoospermia, but they can play a role in combination with other factors. The effects of negative environmental factors are generally reversible with time, typically within three to six months. See Chapter 6 for more details regarding optimizing the environment for sperm production.

- *Hormonal problems.* Abnormal testosterone and estradiol levels can result in significant decreases in sperm production in some circumstances. Also, if the pituitary gland is not sending the right signal to the testicles to make sperm (for example, if FSH levels are under 0.1 IU/L), then azoospermia can result. See "Hormone Testing in Men" in Chapter 4 for more details on hormonal evaluation.

- *Varicoceles.* Dilated veins in the scrotum can be associated with a progressive decrease in sperm production over time. This can lead to complete azoospermia in some men. See "Varicoceles" in Chapter 6 for more information.

- *Chemotherapy or radiation therapy.* Cancer treatments are designed to kill cells that are rapidly dividing. Since cancer cells divide rapidly, chemotherapy and radiation therapy are often an effective treatment. Unfortunately, the cells that make sperm are also rapidly dividing, and therefore are often damaged or killed during the course of cancer treatments. See "Cancer Treatment" in Chapter 6 for more details.

- *Genetic causes.* Some men are born with genetic changes that do not allow their testicles to make sperm. These are typically new mutations that have arisen (because if their fathers had the same mutations, they would not have had children, since currently used techniques for assisted reproduction were not available to them). Current genetic testing options for suspected NOA look at the man's karyotype (all of his chromosomes) for any extra or missing chromosomes, as well as imbalances called translocations, or at the Y chromosome (which only men have), looking for microdeletions, or the absence of certain genes that we know help encode for normal sperm production.

Genetic testing can be done by swabbing the inside of the cheek but are more commonly done with a simple blood test.

Two important caveats about genetics testing. One is that gene therapy is not currently available to treat any genetic abnormalities that may be found. I hope that within the next ten to twenty years scientific research will be able to develop effective gene and stem cell therapy, but as of now these treatments are not possible. The second is that if the results of genetic testing come back as normal, this does not mean that the man does not have a genetic problem; it only means that he does not have a problem that we can test for right now. Scientific research keeps discovering new genes that are involved in sperm production, so in the future we will be able to test for additional genetic abnormalities.

See Chapter 10 for complete details on genetic abnormalities and testing. And see "Management of Non-Obstructive Azoo-spermia" later in this chapter for additional treatment options.

Maturation Arrest

The testicle has two main functions: producing sperm and making testosterone. The Leydig cells are responsible for making testos-terone. The spermatogenic cells and their supporting Sertoli cells (located within the seminiferous tubules) produce sperm. When the spermatogenic cells are not making sperm, this is referred to as testicular failure from a spermatogenic standpoint. Biopsy of testicles with spermatogenic failure typically show one of three pathologic findings:

- *Sertoli cells only (SCO)*. No spermatogenic cells are seen, just the support (Sertoli) cells.

- *Hypospermatogenesis.* Spermatogenic cells are present, but in significantly decreased numbers.

- *Maturation arrest.* Sperm precursor cells are made, but they do not transform into mature sperm.

Men who have only Sertoli cells and men with hypospermato-genesis generally have high FSH levels and smaller testicle volumes. Maturation arrest, however, can be difficult to diagnose. With maturation arrest, immature sperm parts are often being produced in large numbers, so there is lots of activity going on in the testicle, but no fully formed sperm result from it. Since the testicles are being productive (making sperm parts), the brain can be tricked into thinking that the testicular production is good, and therefore the FSH level remains normal. Testicular volume is also often normal since the spermatogenic cells are busy making sperm parts. Because these sperm parts are generally not seen in a semen analysis evaluation and FSH and testicular size are both normal, it is often very difficult to distinguish maturation arrest from obstruction as a cause of azoospermia by using just non-invasive testing. A testicular biopsy is usually needed to find out what is going on; see "Normal FSH and Azoospermia," above. Also see "Management of Non-Obstructive Azoospermia," later in this chapter.

Management of Obstructive Azoospermia

When obstruction is causing azoospermia, there are two main options for men who want to have a biologically related child: surgical reconstruction of the blockage and sperm extraction procedures combined with IVF/ICSI.

Severe sperm transport problems that cannot be reversed can also result in azoospermia that can be managed with similar sperm extraction techniques.

Surgical Reconstruction of Obstructive Azoospermia

Surgical reconstruction options for obstructive azoospermia (OA) depend on the cause and location of the obstruction.

Blockage Involving the Epididymis

Epididymal blockage can be a result of trauma, previous surgery, or congenital abnormalities. Surgical reconstruction (vasoepididymostomy; see Chapter 12) can sometimes be performed if the vas deferens and ejaculatory ducts are otherwise normal and unobstructed.

Blockage Involving the Vas Deferens Within the Scrotum

Vasal blockage, too, can result from trauma, previous surgery, or congenital abnormalities. Surgical reconstruction can be performed if the rest of the vas deferens and ejaculatory ducts are normal. By far the most common reason of obstructive azoospermia is elective vasectomy for contraception. Chapter 12 reviews microsurgical vasectomy reversal techniques, including vasovasostomy and vasoepididymostomy.

Blockage Involving the Inguinal Ring

Inguinal hernia repairs are typically the cause of vasal blockage in this location. Vasal damage at the inguinal ring is very difficult to repair microsurgically due to the location of the obstruction as well as the intensive scar tissue related to the use of mesh in most hernia repairs. Some reports have described attempted repairs with a combined laparoscopic (transabdominal) and scrotal approach, but success rates are relatively low. Sperm extraction combined with IVF/ICSI provides the highest chance of success as well as the least risk of complications in this situation.

Blockage of the Vas Deferens Deep in the Pelvic Region

Blockages deep within the pelvis or retroperitoneum usually are the result of either a previous surgery in the area or a congenital abnormality (such as congenital bilateral absence of the vas deferens; see Chapter 10). These are generally not candidates for surgical reconstruction. Sperm extraction combined with IVF/ICSI usually represents the best approach for these men if they want to have a biologically related child.

Blockage Involving the Ejaculatory Ducts

See "Ejaculatory Duct Obstruction" in Chapter 6.

Sperm Extraction Procedures for Obstructive Azoospermia and Sperm Transport Problems

Efficient and timely transportation of sperm from the testicles to the urethra is an important part of male fertility, and disruption of this process can result in complete azoospermia. When a man has good testicular sperm production but still has no sperm in his ejaculate, then it stands to reason that he has either a blockage (obstructive azoospermia) or a severe sperm transport problem. Examples of obstructive and transport problems include:

- Obstructive problems
  - Vasectomy
  - Ejaculatory duct obstruction
  - Congenital bilateral absence of the vas deferens
  - Congenital blockages, such as bilateral epididymal obstruction
  - Trauma-related obstruction
  - Obstruction related to prior surgery
- Non-obstructive transport problems
  - Failure of emission or ejaculation (e.g., neurologic problems)
  - Acontractile seminal vesicles (e.g., polycystic kidney disease, diabetes)

- Decreased ductal transport of sperm (e.g., from use of alpha blockers or certain antidepressant medications)

Some of these processes are potentially reversible, such as with a vasectomy reversal, resection of ejaculatory duct obstructions, or stopping medications that can inhibit ductal transport of sperm. However, when a reversible cause cannot be readily found or if the treatment fails, then another fertility option is surgical extraction of sperm.

In cases of suspected blockage or sperm transport problems, I always like to check an FSH level. A normal FSH level (1.0–7.0 IU/L) is more than 90 percent accurate in predicting that sperm production is still good, and it suggests that a sperm extraction will be successful.

An important point to remember is that extracted sperm must always be used in conjunction with IVF/ICSI (see Appendix D). A common question is whether extracted sperm can be used with intrauterine insemination, and the answer is no. The extracted sperm are not of a density or maturity to work with IUI, and must be used with IVF/ICSI.

Sperm Extraction Methods

Sperm can be extracted from either the testicle or the epididymis. Techniques involve needle extraction or making a small incision in the scrotum to access the testicle or epididymis.

- Testicular sperm aspiration (TESA) uses a small needle to extract sperm from the testicles.
- Percutaneous epididymal sperm aspiration (PESA) uses a small needle to extract sperm from the epididymis.

- Testicular sperm extraction (TESE) involves making an incision in the scrotum and removing sperm directly from the testicles

- Microepididymal sperm aspiration (MESA) uses a larger incision in the scrotum. The epididymis is then opened under microscopic guidance, after which sperm is extracted.

These extraction procedures can be performed under either local anesthesia alone, local anesthesia with IV sedation, or full general anesthesia.

Fresh Versus Frozen

Sperm can be extracted either fresh at the time of the IVF egg retrieval or at some other time beforehand and then frozen. Once the sperm are frozen, then the woman can start her IVF cycle, with plans for the sperm to be thawed at the time of egg retrieval and injected into each egg. Studies have clearly shown that for men with blockage or transport issues, extracted fresh sperm and frozen sperm have essentially equivalent success rates with IVF. Most people therefore use frozen sperm, as trying to time a fresh sperm extraction with an egg retrieval can be difficult. During an IVF cycle the exact date that the woman's eggs are going to be ready for retrieval is not known until a few days beforehand. This makes trying to time a simultaneous extraction for the male a challenge, since sperm extraction requires the coordination of a procedure room and any necessary staff, as well as making sure that the lab has time set aside to properly process the extracted tissue. By extracting and freezing the sperm before starting the IVF cycle, the date and time of the procedure can be planned so that there are no problems with the availability of the surgeon, procedure room, anesthesia, and lab. In addition, by extracting the sperm beforehand, the man and the woman are not simultaneously undergoing procedures, so they can help each other out during the recovery process. The presence of sperm can also be confirmed prior to starting an expensive IVF cycle. There is no rush to use frozen sperm; once it is frozen it can be used successfully years later if needed, without a significant loss in its fertility potential.

Testicular Sperm Versus Epididymal Sperm

Studies have shown that for men with sperm blockage or transport problems, IVF success rates are equivalent for sperm extracted from the testicle and sperm extracted from the epididymis. Some labs prefer to use epididymal sperm, since these tend to have more immediate motility and therefore it can be easier to identify live sperm. However, other labs feel that testicular sperm tend to survive the freeze-and-thaw process better than epididymal sperm. The other advantage of testicular sperm is that newly made sperm are being extracted, whereas the sperm from the blocked epididymal region can contain higher numbers of stagnant sperm that have been sitting around trapped in the epididymis for a long time waiting to be reabsorbed by the body. Studies in men with blockages have shown higher rates of elevated sperm DNA fragmentation in epididymal sperm in comparison to testicular sperm.

Recommendations

For men with sperm obstruction or transport problems, I prefer to perform TESA procedures under IV sedation and freeze the sperm for later use.

One reason I prefer TESA is that the nerve supply to the testicle is clustered around the epididymis, making the epididymal area generally the most sensitive part of the scrotal contents for most men. Therefore, retrieving sperm from the testicle avoids the sensitive epididymis and can potentially decrease discomfort. I also prefer to extract testicular sperm, since the labs that I work with feel that they survive the freeze-and-thaw process better than epididymal sperm. There is good evidence as well that the fresher testicular sperm may be healthier than the potentially stagnant epididymal sperm. Even though IVF success rates have been shown to be comparable between epididymal and testicular sperm, higher rates of sperm DNA fragmentation are found in epididymal sperm in men with blockages, so I prefer to retrieve freshly made testicular sperm for use with IVF.

I like the needle extraction (TESA) technique, since it minimizes trauma to the testicle. Recovery times are faster if an incision is not needed, which is possible at least 90 percent of the time. In less than 10 percent of TESA cases, the testicular tubules are of a thicker consistency and so are very difficult to draw up into the needle; consequently a small incision may be needed to retrieve sperm from the testicle.

Most men are nervous about having a procedure on their scrotum, and that nervousness can translate into a tight scrotum, which can make the procedure more difficult and more uncomfortable. By using IV sedation provided by trained anesthesia personnel, the patient remains safe, relaxed, and comfortable throughout the procedure.

Using the TESA technique in men with normal sperm production, I am almost always able to get enough sperm for multiple IVF cycles, so if more than one IVF cycle is needed, the man does not have to go through the extraction procedure again. My goal is generally to extract enough for three vials of frozen sperm, with the labs I generally work with defining one vial as sufficient for one fresh IVF cycle. In my experience, PESA usually extracts less sperm, and therefore fewer vials can be frozen for future IVF cycles. The MESA procedure typically extracts lots of sperm, so multiple backup frozen vials can be obtained. However, the MESA procedure also tends to be very invasive, requiring a large scrotal incision, and it is more expensive. In my experience, TESA is well tolerated, minimally invasive, and significantly less expensive. It requires less anesthesia, has a shorter recovery time, does not damage the epididymis (see below), and yields enough sperm for multiple IVF cycles.

Men who have had a previous vasectomy often choose to do a sperm extraction and IVF/ICSI instead of a vasectomy reversal. Most of these men have good results and high chances of pregnancy with this procedure as long as the female partner is a good candidate for IVF. However, a few times a year I get a couple who has had a successful sperm extraction but then did not have a good experience with IVF (for example, the woman did not respond well to the IVF medications or had significant complications, such as hyperstimulation). These couples often come back asking if a reversal is still a possible option. If TESA has been performed, then there is minimal extra scar tissue in the scrotum and the epididymis is still intact, so vasectomy reversal rates should not be negatively impacted by the prior extraction procedure. However, if an epididymal sperm extraction was performed initially, then this significantly increases the risk that obstructing scar tissue may be present within the epididymis (especially if MESA was used). This epididymal damage can increase the chances that a vas-to-epididymis reversal connection will be needed (which is less optimal in terms of success rates) or that a microsurgical reconstruction might not even be able to be performed (see Chapter 12).Of course, other male fertility experts may prefer a different sperm extraction approach for IVF/ICSI.

Management of Non-Obstructive Azoospermia

The first step in managing non-obstructive azoospermia (NOA) is to identify and treat any reversible causes that could be contributing to the sperm production problem. These include all of the general interventions that are reviewed in Chapters 4 through 6.

Sometimes sperm counts can be restored to good levels, such as in men who have been taking exogenous androgens. Pregnancy with natural intercourse or low-tech treatments from the female side (clomiphene, insemination, etc.) are often successful for these couples. If small amounts of sperm return to the ejaculate, then the semen will need to be evaluated to make sure enough sperm are present to proceed with IVF/ICSI (see "Virtual Azoospermia" earlier in this chapter).

However, for men in whom all reversible factors have been treated but who still remain azoospermic, genetic testing is indicated, along with genetic counseling if appropriate—see Chapter 10. In this situation, fertility options include adoption, the use of donor sperm with IUI (see Appendix F), the use of donor embryos, and sperm extraction combined with IVF/ICSI.

Sperm Extraction for NOA

Some men with non-obstructive azoospermia have small "islands" of sperm production that exist within the testicles but simply do not produce enough sperm to spill over into the ejaculate. In these cases, it may be possible to extract small amounts of sperm from the testicles for use with IVF/ICSI. To find usable sperm in men with NOA, different techniques of testicular sperm extraction need to be used instead of those employed for men with obstructive azoo-spermia.

Many couples in whom the male partner is found to have non-obstructive azoospermia choose either adoption, the use of donor embryos, or donor sperm combined with intrauterine insemination. Men with NOA who wish to explore their chances of having a child who is biologically related to them need to consider a few issues. If there is no obvious reason for the NOA (such as previous chemotherapy or radiation therapy, exogenous testosterone use, etc.), then most likely there is a genetic basis for the sperm production problem. Some of these genetic problems can be uncovered by currently available tests (see Chapter 10). However, if genetic testing comes back normal, this does not mean that a genetic abnormality is not present, but only that the man does not have a genetic problem that science can currently test for. Either way, it should be assumed that genetic sperm production problems will most likely be passed on to any male offspring, who would then be expected to have similar sperm production problems. By the time these offspring are old enough to have children themselves, new gene or stem cell therapies may be available. However, this might not be the case, and couples must be comfortable with passing on this potential genetic legacy to future generations. Genetic counseling is sometimes helpful for couples facing these tough decisions, as discussed in Chapter 10.

Genetic testing may also provide prognostic information on the chances of finding sperm by testicular sperm extraction. If Y chromosome microdeletions involving the AZFa and/or AZFb regions are found, then any attempts at testicular sperm extraction will generally not be successful. However, if an AZFc deletion or another type of genetic problem (including Klinefelter's disease) is discovered, then the man may be a candidate for testicular sperm extraction. See Chapter 10 for more details on genetic testing.

Prior to any attempted sperm extraction procedure in NOA men, the environment for sperm production should be fully optimized in order to improve the odds of a successful sperm extraction (see Chapters 4 through 6). There is also a chance that with some intervention, small numbers of sperm might return to the ejaculate, allowing them to be used for IVF/ICSI without having to perform an extraction procedure. Potential interventions include:

- Treating low testosterone levels (at a minimum testosterone levels should be 300 ng/dL, and ideally higher)
- Treatment of clinically significant varicoceles
- Lifestyle changes (e.g., avoiding hot tubs and saunas, stopping smoking, etc.)
- Modification of medications that might be detrimental to sperm production

Once the environment for sperm production has been optimized, several choices need to be made, including the type of surgical sperm extraction procedure that will be performed and whether the sperm are going to be extracted at the same time as the woman's egg retrieval or if the sperm extraction is going to be performed first, with the woman proceeding with IVF only if sperm are found at the time of the extraction.

Types of Extraction Procedures for NOA

Standard Testicular Sperm Aspiration (TESA)

The TESA procedure involves a needle aspiration of testicular tubules and is 90–95 percent successful in retrieving sperm in men with obstructive azoospermia, such as in post-vasectomy patients. However, the standard TESA procedure does not achieve a good sampling of multiple different areas of the testicle, which is necessary for finding the small islands of sperm production in men with NOA. Success rates of finding sperm in NOA men with use of a standard TESA procedure on one side are typically around 10–20 percent.

Upper/Middle/Lower Pole Biopsy

Testicular sperm extraction (TESE) is the procedure used when sperm are extracted through an incision in the scrotum (as opposed to TESA, which involves a needle aspiration and no incision). Performing a TESE or TESA of the upper pole, middle pole, and lower pole of each testicle allows better sampling than the standard single site TESA procedure. Some studies have reported success rates of up to 45 percent with these TESE procedures, but I have found them typically to yield lower success rates (25–30 percent) in finding sperm. This procedure can be performed under local anesthesia, IV sedation, or general anesthesia.

Microscopic Testicular Sperm Extraction (mTESE)

In the mTESE procedure, the testicle is carefully opened widely and the tubules are thoroughly examined using an operating micro-scope. Small areas of dilated tubules can sometimes be seen, and these often contain viable sperm. Success rates have been reported to be as high as 50–65 percent in some studies, although most studies report a 40–55 percent success rate in men without AZFa or AZFb microdeletions on the Y chromosome. Microscopic testicular sperm extraction is generally performed on an outpatient basis under general anesthesia. Due to the more invasive nature of the mTESE procedure, some degree of testicular damage can occur. Studies have shown that about 5–10 percent of men undergoing mTESE need to have testosterone replacement started after the procedure.

Fine-Needle Mapping of the Testicle

Mapping the testicle using fine-needle aspiration (FNA) involves a two-part procedure. The first part (the actual mapping portion) is performed under local anesthesia or IV sedation and involves taking ten to fifteen small biopsies from each testicle using a very thin needle. This type of needle retrieves just enough tissue for analysis but is small enough that it does not significantly damage the testicle. The extracted tissue is then placed on separate glass slides and evaluated by a pathologist for the presence of sperm. The location of each extracted piece of tissue is labeled and tracked so that if sperm are found on that slide, the surgeon knows exactly which area of the testicle that sperm came from. Excellent sampling of all parts of the testicles can be safely accomplished. However, all of the extracted tissue is placed on glass slides and stained for analysis, so any sperm that are found are not usable for IVF/ICSI. If sperm are identified, then a second procedure is needed to go back to the place where they were found and retrieve more for use in IVF/ICSI. This process typically involves a focused mTESE that looks only at the areas of the testicle where sperm were seen by the FNA sampling. Success rates of FNA mapping combined with mTESE are comparable to mTESE used alone. Advantages of this procedure include that if no sperm are seen on any of the FNA samples, then the man is spared the more invasive mTESE procedure and the woman does not needlessly start an expensive IVF cycle. Studies have shown that if a man with NOA has no sperm found on an FNA mapping procedure, that the chance of finding sperm on a subsequent mTESE is less than 3–5 percent. The disadvantage of the FNA mapping is that in order to successfully retrieve usable sperm, two surgeries are necessary instead of one. Also, there is a small chance (about 15 percent) that when small numbers of sperm are found at the time of the mapping, the subsequent mTESE procedure will not be successful in retrieving usable sperm.

Repeated Sperm Extractions

It is generally recommended that if a man is going to have a repeat sperm extraction on the same testicle, six months should pass between the extraction attempts. This allows the testicle time to heal and can potentially increase the chance of finding sperm. However, with the mapping procedure, the needles used for FNA are so small that minimal testicular damage occurs and subsequent mTESE does not need to be delayed.

Fresh vs. Frozen Sperm for IVF/ICSI with Non-Obstructive Azoospermia

In general, the chance of finding sperm in men with non-obstructive azoospermia using the latest extraction techniques (mTESE and FNA mapping) is around 40–55 percent. Since sperm are not going to be found in at least half of men with NOA, some couples find it appealing to do a sperm extraction first to see if sperm are even present before proceeding with an expensive IVF cycle. However, the topic of using fresh versus frozen sperm for IVF in men with NOA is an area of great debate.

Significant controversy exists as to whether IVF/ICSI success rates are improved when freshly extracted sperm is used from men with NOA, as opposed to frozen sperm. Leading experts in the field regularly debate the subject, so far with no definitive answer. Some studies have shown improved rates of success with fresh sperm, while others show equivalent rates of success using fresh or frozen sperm. My overall opinion is that it is not clear that fresh sperm from men with NOA will have superior IVF outcomes compared with frozen sperm in cases where enough viable sperm are available to use. However, I feel that using fresh sperm increases the chances that enough sperm will be available to inject all of the available eggs retrieved for an IVF cycle. This is because when sperm go through the freeze-and-thaw process, generally around 50–75 percent of the sperm do not survive even in the best of circumstances (with lower percentages of sperm surviving from samples with very low starting numbers of sperm). For IVF/ICSI, typically only about five to twenty live sperm are needed, since this is usually the number of eggs retrieved from the woman. In men with obstructive azoospermia, the number of extracted sperm is generally quite large (several thousand sperm), so if 50–75 percent of them do not survive cryopreservation and thawing, plenty of viable sperm are still left over. However, in men with NOA, usually only a very small number of sperm are retrieved with an extraction procedure. Using current cryopreservation techniques on these very small numbers of sperm means that when it comes time to thaw them out for use, no viable sperm are available up to two-thirds of the time. Clearly, better laboratory freezing techniques are needed, and I am hopeful that ongoing research in this field will deliver better outcomes in the future.

The other significant consideration when trying to decide whether to use fresh or frozen sperm for IVF in men with NOA is the issue of procedure scheduling. If fresh sperm are to be used, trying to coordinate a fresh testicular sperm extraction with the time of a woman's egg retrieval can be difficult from a logistical standpoint. When a woman is undergoing an IVF cycle, she is being constantly monitored to determine the exact time when her eggs will be ready for retrieval. The IVF lab will generally aim for a three-day window in which the eggs will most likely be ready for retrieval, but the exact day will not be known until a few days prior. These retrieved eggs must then be injected with sperm within a fairly narrow time frame, around six hours, so any sperm retrieval procedure must be closely coordinated with the time of the egg retrieval if fresh sperm are going to be used. Most sperm extraction procedures for NOA are quite long (more than two hours), and trying to find operating room time for such lengthy procedures with only a few days' notice is often difficult, if not impossible, in many places. Surgery centers are usually booked weeks to months ahead of time and cannot hold open blocks of time that span several days. Hospitals have more flexibility, but non-emergency surgical cases that are added on at the last minute are often pushed late into the evening, when the IVF labs (which are needed to evaluate and process the sperm) are no longer open. Hospital facility fees are also often extremely high for these procedures, which are usually not covered by insurance. The other factor to consider is the extremely important role of the fertility lab in being able to successfully find sperm in NOA men. Specialized laboratory personnel must devote a large amount of time to thoroughly processing and searching through the extracted tissue to find whatever sperm may be there, if any. The uncertain nature of trying to coordinate the extraction with the time of the egg retrieval often leaves the lab unable to devote as much time as they would like for properly processing the extracted tissue.

Egg Vitrification

If timing a sperm extraction with an IVF cycle is difficult and small numbers of sperm do not freeze well, what about freezing (vitrifying) eggs? That way, the woman can go through an IVF cycle and have her eggs retrieved and frozen. The man can then have a scheduled mTESE on an elective basis when the full attention of the IVF lab embryologists can be focused on looking for sperm in the extracted tissue. If sperm are found, then frozen eggs can be thawed and injected. If no sperm are found, then the couple may choose to inject the eggs with donor sperm at a later time.

Until recently, unfertilized eggs did not freeze well (as opposed to embryos, which are routinely frozen and used later with good outcomes). However, new freezing techniques now allow successful egg freezing. Some encouraging preliminary studies have suggested that pregnancy rates using vitrified eggs for IVF were similar to those using fresh eggs. However, the field of egg vitrification is quite new, and some IVF lab directors question whether these early positive studies are applicable to the IVF population as a whole. I have heard estimates of up to a 20 percent decrease in expected pregnancy rates with the use of vitrified eggs, although these numbers will need to be evaluated further with future well-designed research trials. What is clear is that egg freezing technology has made great strides and opens up another potential option for couples with NOA.

Donor Sperm Backup

Any time there is a question of whether enough sperm are going to be present at the time of egg retrieval, it's a good idea to consider having donor sperm backup. Any eggs that are not fertilized by the patient's sperm can then be injected with the donor sperm. This strategy allows for a backup plan in situations where otherwise there may be limited options left for conception. See Appendix F for more details on donor sperm.

Pros and Cons of Various Approaches

As detailed above, there are several options for men with NOA who want to attempt testicular sperm extraction, all of which have positives and negatives associated with them.

Use of Frozen Extracted Sperm with Donor Sperm Backup

Positives:

- The sperm extraction can be performed on an elective basis, allowing the IVF lab to plan for adequate staffing. This permits them to fully process and evaluate the extracted tissue in an ideal setting

- If sperm are not found (there is up to a 55–60 percent chance of this), then an unnecessary, expensive IVF procedure can be avoided.

Negatives:

- Up to two-thirds of men with small amounts of sperm successfully extracted will still not have viable sperm upon thawing of the specimens. This risk can be mitigated by having donor sperm backup available.

Fresh Sperm Extraction Timed with Fresh Egg Retrieval

Positives:

- Any sperm that are found do not need to be frozen.
- Retrieved eggs do not need to be frozen.

Negatives:

- Coordination of the extraction procedure with the exact day of egg retrieval can be very difficult.
- Uncertainty as to egg retrieval date can mean that the IVF lab will not have enough staff available to optimally process the tissue obtained with sperm extraction.
- There is up to a 55–60 percent chance that sperm may not be found, and therefore an expensive IVF cycle will have been performed needlessly. This risk can be mitigated by having donor sperm backup.

Egg Retrieval and Vitrification (Freezing) Followed by Fresh mTESE

Positives:

- Any sperm that are found do not need to be frozen.
- The sperm extraction can be performed on an elective basis, with the IVF lab being able to plan for adequate staffing to fully process and evaluate the extracted tissue.

Negatives:

- The need to freeze the eggs, which may decrease pregnancy rates by up to 20 percent (though this is controversial).
- Up to a 55–60 percent chance that sperm will not found, and therefore an expensive IVF cycle will have been performed

needlessly. This risk can be mitigated by having donor sperm backup.

Recommendations

I feel that the literature best supports the use of mTESE to produce fresh sperm timed with an IVF/ICSI cycle as the "gold standard" for optimizing the chances of finding usable sperm. The FNA mapping procedure prior to the mTESE is also a good option, with the advantage of potentially avoiding the more expensive mTESE and IVF procedures in over half of cases. The disadvantage of the FNA mapping is that two scrotal procedures (instead of one) are needed to obtain usable sperm, so some couples choose to just proceed straight to mTESE.

As mentioned previously, it is difficult to schedule a mTESE procedure to produce fresh sperm in conjunction with a woman's egg retrieval. However, multiple centers around the country have a great enough volume of mTESE cases that they are able to set aside several periods a year for these short-notice situations. An example of one such center is Cornell Medical Center in New York City with Dr. Peter Schlegal, who invented the mTESE procedure. Dr. Schlegal performs such a large number of these procedures that several times a year he schedules a week where he does nothing but mTESEs. During these weeks, all of the female partners of the men with NOA are cycled so that their eggs will be ready for retrieval sometime during that week. Dr. Schlegal has an operating room ready and waiting the entire week, so that when a woman's eggs are ready, he can immediately take the male partner in for his mTESE procedure. During that week, the IVF lab brings in extra embryology personnel so that the lab is ready at any time for processing of the testicular specimens. It is with this type of setup that Dr. Schlegal is able to find sperm in up to 55 percent of the men with NOA that he sees. Of course, because this center is in New

York City, the procedure is quite expensive, currently costing around \$30,000–35,000 for the mTESE (this includes the cost of the IVF/ICSI, but not travel and hotel expenses).

Dr. Schlegal's unique setup is difficult to replicate, although some facilities around the country have been able to devise a successful coordination strategy for mTESE procedures producing fresh sperm timed with egg retrieval for IVF. If you are considering having mTESE done with the aim of producing fresh sperm, I recommend that you first address a few specific questions with your doctor:

- Be sure to carefully question your surgeon about how he or she plans to schedule a procedure that can take two hours or more with only a few days' notice. Is the facility going to be able to provide adequate operating time? Is it going to be rushed by being squeezed in between other scheduled cases? Is the procedure likely to start at 6:30 p.m., when the surgeon might be not be fully rested for such a demanding, several-hour microsurgical procedure?
- Talk with the IVF lab and make sure that they are going to be able to coordinate their schedule so that they will have enough available personnel at the time of the procedure to thoroughly process and evaluate the extracted tissue.
- See what the exact facility cost for the extraction procedure is going to be, especially if it is going to be at a hospital.

I personally prefer to start with an FNA mapping procedure, because in over 50 percent of NOA couples, no sperm will be found and the cost and risks of both a more invasive mTESE procedure and IVF can be avoided. Where I practice, surgery center and lab personnel availability makes it difficult to coordinate mTESE with an IVF cycle so that both sperm and egg can be used fresh. In addition, I prefer not to freeze sperm that have been successfully extracted from men with NOA. Therefore, if sperm are found on the mapping procedure, then I discuss with the couple the option of having mTESE performed by one of my colleagues who practices in an area where mTESE can be scheduled to provide fresh sperm optimally coordinated with the IVF/ICSI cycle. These centers are usually in academic institutions, where the surgeons often have flexible administrative or research time that they can utilize to increase their availability for these short-notice procedures.

10

Genetics

Genetics is an exciting and rapidly developing field that is trans-
forming our understanding of the body and how to treat disease.
The genes contained in our chromosomes encode the building
instructions for every cell in our body, so it is not surprising that
genetic problems can interfere with male fertility. Genetic abnormalities are found at a much higher rate in men having fertility
problems, with various studies finding an eight- to hundredfold
increased risk of genetic problems in this population of men.
Genetic abnormalities can impact fertility in three ways: an inability
to conceive a pregnancy, an elevated risk of early pregnancy loss,
and a risk of transmitting genetic abnormalities to biologically
related children.

A Review of Basic Genetics

Humans normally have forty-six chromosomes (twenty-three pairs
of chromosomes). Forty-four of the chromosomes are what are
called autosomes, and two are the sex chromosomes, which can be
either an X chromosome or a Y chromosome. Women have two X
chromosomes (XX), and men have one X and one Y (XY). A
person's karyotype is the number and structure of his or her
chromosomes. A person's phenotype is his or her observable

physical characteristics, which result when the person's genes interact with the environment.

When sperm and eggs are produced by males and females, respectively, the chromosomes split so that each sperm or each egg receives twenty-three chromosomes. When fertilization occurs, the egg and sperm from each partner combine, and each contribute its twenty-three chromosomes to provide the resulting embryo with the full set of forty-six chromosomes. The Y chromosome, if present, makes that embryo become male.

There are two important, distinct areas on the Y chromosome that we know impact male fertility:

- *SRY (sex-determining region Y) gene.* Normally present on the Y chromosome, this gene makes the fetus become a phenotypic male—that is, the child looks anatomically like a male. If the SRY gene is not present, the child will look anatomically like a female.

- *AZF (azoospermic factor) region of genes.* This region is important for normal sperm production. If it is missing (called a Y chromosome microdeletion), these men usually have little or no sperm production.

Causes of Genetic Problems

Genetic problems can occur in one of two ways: through spontaneous gene mutations or by inheriting an abnormal gene from one of the parents. Many genetic problems are clearly inherited from the parents, such as the cystic fibrosis gene. However, not all genetic problems affecting sperm production are passed from generation to generation. Men with extremely low sperm counts are sometimes confused as to how they can have a genetic sperm production problem when their father (and often their siblings as well) have had no problems conceiving children. The reason is that many of these genetic male-factor problems result from spontaneous new mutations. If their fathers had had the same genetic problem, then the patient likely would not have been conceived, since many of the current high-tech fertility options were largely not available to the previous generation (the first successful IVF cycle was in 1978).

New mutations can arise within a man's chromosomes via several mechanisms:

- *Deletions.* Genes can be deleted from chromosomes for many different reasons, including abnormalities that occur during cell division.

- *Translocations.* Genetic translocations occur when genetic material is exchanged abnormally between a person's chromosomes. No genetic material is lost during this rearrangement, so the person with the translocation typically does not have any other apparent health problems. However, when the chromosomes are split up during egg or sperm formation, sometimes the egg or sperm can end up with too much or too little genetic information. Depending on the translocation type, this can result in an increased risk of miscarriage, chromosomal abnormalities (such as Down syndrome), and certain types of cancer or other health problems.

- *Inversions.* Similar to translocations, inversions do not involve the loss of genetic material in the parent. Rather, there is a rearrangement of the order of the genes within a chromosome. Again, this typically does not impact the parent as much as it can affect offspring, since during sperm formation the amount of DNA that each sperm receives might be unbalanced.

Genetic Counseling

Genetic counselors are clinical specialists who are trained in evaluating genetic abnormalities and discussing their potential consequences with patients. They are often found working in children's hospitals, since this is the population in which the majority of genetic problems are diagnosed, but they regularly work with adults too.

Patients who have a karyotype abnormality should have genetic counseling. This can help to determine the odds that their genetic problems will impact their own fertility or the health of their offspring. In addition, genetic counselors can provide valuable information about general health concerns associated with certain genetic problems, such as Klinefelter's disease. Men with Y chromosome microdeletions do not necessarily need formal genetic counseling if they are working with a male fertility specialist, since these problems do not generally impact other areas of their health besides reproduction. However, these patients need to know that if their own sperm are used, then any resulting male offspring will harbor these same microdeletions.

Genetic Testing

Currently, there are four main genetic tests that can be performed in men with fertility problems:

- *Karyotype testing.* Evaluates the chromosomes for problems resulting from deletions, translocations, and inversions.

- *Y chromosome microdeletion (YCMD) testing.* Looks for specific deletions in the AZF region of the Y chromosome that are known to encode for sperm production

- *Cystic fibrosis testing.* Men who carry two copies of the cystic fibrosis gene can have sperm blockage problems (congenital bilateral absence of the vas deferens, CBAVD), as well as the disease cystic fibrosis.

- *Sperm DNA testing.* Evaluates the integrity of the sperm DNA itself.

The field of genetics is rapidly evolving, and new genes are being discovered every year. Although the genes of the AZF region are extremely important, there are certainly many more genes involved in maintaining normal sperm production, and most of these have not yet been identified and so cannot yet be tested for. Therefore, if genetic testing results on a man come back as normal, this does not completely rule out the presence of genetic problem; it merely means that the man does not have any genetic abnormalities that we can test for at this time.

The other factor to keep in mind is that there are currently no gene therapies or embryonic stem cell treatments that can correct fertility-related genetic abnormalities. The value of a genetic test must therefore be weighed against the financial costs of that test. Factors to consider when deciding whether to proceed with genetic testing include:

- Cost of the test (and insurance coverage). See Appendix C for a listing of the costs of genetic testing if it is not covered by insurance.
- How important it is to a particular couple that they may be passing on possible genetic abnormalities to their offspring. Remember, genetic abnormalities that we cannot yet test for can be passed on as well.
- Any potential impact that the findings might have on future treatment options.
- The potential impact that a genetic abnormality (such as Klinefelter's) can have on a person's overall health.

Karyotype and Y Chromosome Microdeletion Testing

Currently, the established fertility guidelines recommend karyotype and Y chromosome microdeletion genetic testing for men with a sperm count of under 5 million/cc and no other known significant causes of infertility (such as obstruction or previous chemotherapy, among others). However, genetic testing can be expensive, and in some men with relatively low sperm counts, the chance of finding a genetic abnormality with current testing capabilities is very low. A cost-benefit analysis therefore needs to be made for each couple as to whether the genetic information they can obtain from genetic testing has the potential to be useful enough to justify its cost.

In general, men with no sperm in the ejaculate (azoospermia) who have no blockage issues have about a 15–20 percent chance of having genetic testing show an abnormal karyotype or Y chromosome microdeletion. In contrast, men with oligospermia (low sperm count) have only a 5–6 percent chance of having a genetic abnormality found upon testing.

In a recently published paper, the Cleveland Clinic evaluated costs and benefits and concluded that a better cutoff for ordering genetic testing would be a density of 2.5 million sperm/cc or under. This is the criteria that I currently use in my practice, since I almost never find that genetic testing is useful in men with sperm densities of between 2.5 and 5 million/cc. An exception to this general rule is found in men whose partners have had unexplained recurrent pregnancy loss. In this situation, I will often order a karyotype test in the male partner (regardless of his sperm count), since translocations and inversions may contribute to pregnancy loss in men with fairly high sperm counts.

Cystic Fibrosis Screening

The CFTR (cystic fibrosis transmembrane conductance regulator) gene is associated with cystic fibrosis. CFTR testing is indicated in two circumstances: if there is concern about a congenital vasal abnormality, or if the female partner is found to be a cystic fibrosis gene carrier, in order to assess the risk of any subsequent children developing the disease.

Otherwise, if a man has sperm in the ejaculate and no suspected genital duct structural abnormality (such as a non-palpable vas deferens on one side), then CFTR testing is not indicated.

Sperm DNA Testing

The integrity of sperm DNA can be assessed by looking at the ability of sperm DNA to resist fragmentation. Indications for sperm DNA testing include:

- Normal semen analysis but unexplained persistent infertility
- Recurrent unexplained pregnancy loss
- ˙Recurrent unexplained IVF failure

Some clinicians also use sperm DNA testing to assess the integrity of sperm DNA in various at-risk men, such as those who have had prior chemotherapy or those considered to be of advanced paternal age (although no official guidelines have been established for these groups of patients). See Chapter 11 for more detailed information about sperm DNA testing.

Karyotype-Related Genetic Abnormalities

Potential abnormalities that can be detected with karyotype testing include:

- Klinefelter's disease
- 46 XX syndrome
- 47 XYY syndrome
- Translocations and inversions, both of which can lead to an increased risk of recurrent pregnancy loss

I generally use ICD-9 code 257.9 (testicular failure) as the diagnosis code for karyotype testing, but code 606.9 (male infertility) can also be used if you have coverage for infertility testing. Beginning in October 2015, the new ICD-10 codes to use will be E29.9 (testicular failure) and N46.9 (male infertility).

See Appendix C for the cost of karyotype testing if it is not covered by insurance.

Klinefelter's Disease

Klinefelter's is the most common karyotype abnormality in male fertility. This genetic abnormality is cause by having an extra X chromosome, and therefore these men have forty-seven chromosomes (instead of forty-six), with two X chromosomes and one Y chromosome (instead of one X and one Y). Another way to express it is that men with Klinefelter's have a 47 XXY karyotype (normal for a male is 46 XY). Klinefelter's affects one in five hundred live male births and is the cause of 14 percent of cases of nonobstructive azoospermia. One known risk factor for developing Klinefelter's is increased maternal age.

Presentation

Classic findings seen in men with Klinefelter's disease include:

- Small, firm testes
- Gynecomastia (enlargement of breast tissue)
- Azoospermia (a small percentage of men with Klinefelter's have small amounts of sperm in the ejaculate)

Men with Klinefelter's often also have delayed or decreased development of secondary sexual characteristics, such as body and facial hair and muscle development.

Other common findings include:

- Tall stature
- Obesity
- Eunuchoid body proportions (lower body segment longer than upper body, arm span 5 cm or more longer than height)

However, there is very wide variation between men with Klinefelter's disease. "Classic" Klinefelter's patients are often diagnosed at a younger age, as there is usually a lack of development of normal secondary sexual characteristics at puberty. However, many men with Klinefelter's appear completely normal with the exception of having small, firm testicles. These men can experience fairly normal pubertal changes and are diagnosed only as adults when they attempt to have children.

Men with Klinefelter's generally have:

- Elevated FSH levels
- Elevated LH levels
- Low testosterone levels

Approximately 5–10 percent of men with Klinefelter's also have Y chromosome microdeletions.

Men with Klinefelter's are at an increased risk of other general health problems, so they need to have a primary care physician who is familiar with the potential medical problems associated with a 47 XXY karyotype. These include an increased risk of:

- Diabetes
- Extragonadal germ cell tumors
- Leukemia
- Breast cancer (mean age of diagnosis is sixty-five years)
- Non-Hodgkin's lymphoma

- Osteoporosis (possibly in combination with vitamin D deficiency)
- Clotting abnormalities, such as deep venous thrombosis or pulmonary embolism
- Adrenal gland insufficiency
- Lung cancer
- Mitral valve prolapse
- History of undescended testicles (in up to 10–25 percent of men)

It's important to remember that despite the increased risk of certain forms of cancer in these men, the majority of them do not develop those malignancies.

I do recommend genetic counseling for all men with a diagnosis of Klinefelter's disease. General health maintenance recommendations include:

- Monitoring of labs, including testosterone, estradiol, cortisol, hematocrit, TSH, and vitamin D
- DEXA scan to evaluate for osteoporosis
- Echocardiogram to look for mitral valve prolapse

Fertility Options

Almost all men with Klinefelter's have azoospermia. Options for fatherhood include:

- Adoption
- Intrauterine insemination with donor sperm
- Donor embryos
- Attempted sperm extraction combined with IVF/ICSI

Note: In some circumstances (10–15 percent of the time), a man with Klinefelter's can have a condition called mosaicism, in which a certain percentage of his body cells have a 47 XXY karyotype and the rest are normal 46 XY. These men typically have higher testosterone levels and larger testicle sizes. Many of these men are still azoospermic, but approximately 50 percent have very small amounts of sperm in the ejaculate (an average of about 4 to 5 million sperm per cc).

Sperm can sometimes be found in the testicles of azoospermic men with Klinefelter's (or mosaic Klinefelter's) and used successfully with IVF/ICSI. Microscopic testicular sperm extraction (mTESE) is generally used due to its relatively high success rates in finding sperm; see "Management of Non-Obstructive Azoospermia" in Chapter 9). Prior to undergoing mTESE, the man's testosterone level should be raised to greater than 250 ng/dL using medications such as anastrazole. This will improve the chances of finding sperm. Y chromosome microdeletion testing is also recommended, since approximately 5–10 percent of men with Klinefelter's also have YCMDs.

Centers using mTESE in men with Klinefelter's disease have had success rates of 40–70 percent in terms of finding enough sperm for a fresh cycle of IVF/ICSI. Most sperm that are surgically retrieved are genetically normal. Supposedly, the use of extracted sperm has not resulted in the live birth of any children with Klinefelter's, but a few aborted fetuses have shown genetic abnormalities. Some centers recommend the use of preimplantation genetic diagnosis (PGD) due to the increased risk of aneuploidy (an abnormal number of chromosomes) in the embryos.

Y Chromosome Microdeletions

Only men have a Y chromosome, and the genes that encode for normal sperm production are found on this chromosome. Therefore, deletions on the Y chromosome can have a profound impact on semen parameters if they affect the genes that control sperm production. The AZF (azoospermic factor) region has been found to play a very important role in sperm production. It is divided into three sections:

- AZFa (also called DYS273 and DYS275, or P5/proxP1 by some labs)
- AZFb (also called DYS209 and DYS224, or P5/distP1 by some labs)
- AZFc (also called DAZ and SPGY, or b2/b4 by some labs)

Deletions in the AZF region are found in 6–14 percent of men with severe oligospermia and in 3–18 percent of men with complete azoospermia. The impact on sperm production depends on which of the AZF sections is missing:

- AZFa deletion, which results in a severe production problem causing complete azoospermia, is found in about 1 percent of azoospermic men
- AZFb deletion, which also results in a severe production problem causing complete azoospermia, is found in about 1–2 percent of azoospermic men
- AZFc deletion, which results in a slightly less severe production problems, is found in up to 13 percent of azoospermic men and 6–14 percent of men with severe oligospermia

The ICD-9 diagnosis code for YCMD testing is 257.9 (testicular failure), but code 606.9 (male infertility) can also be used if you have infertility testing coverage. Beginning in October 2015, the new ICD-10 codes to use will be E29.9 (testicular failure) and N46.9 (male infertility).

See Appendix C for the cost of YCMD testing if it is not covered by insurance.

Fertility Options

In men with an AZFa or AZFb deletion, there is no sperm production at all, and attempted testicular sperm extraction will not be successful; adoption, donor sperm, and donor embryos are the only options for having a child. Approximately 40–55 percent of men with only AZFc deletions can have small islands of sperm production that can be found by sperm extraction techniques (such as mTESE) and used in conjunction with IVF/ICSI; see "Management of Non-Obstructive Azoospermia" in Chapter 9).

Genetic Implications

Y chromosome microdeletions (YCMDs) are not yet known to be associated with significant health problems, other than potentially lower testosterone levels and a possible increased risk of testicular cancer. However, it must be remembered that if sperm are used from a man with YCMDs, then those same YCMDs are going to be passed on to any male children the couple conceives, presumably resulting in similar testicular function problems for those boys. By the time these male children reach reproductive age, there may be new, innovative treatments available (such as gene or stem cell therapy), but this is by no means guaranteed.

Cystic Fibrosis

Cystic fibrosis (CF) is a severe respiratory disease that can also affect the function of the liver, pancreas, and intestines. CF patients have thick mucus secretions that lead to recurrent lung infections, and in the past, few people with CF lived to reproductive age. However, with the advent of better antibiotics and respiratory care, CF patients are living much longer, healthier, and more productive lives.

The CFTR (CF transmembrane conductance regulator) gene is responsible for the movement of electrolytes out of the cells. If the CFTR gene is not working, then water does not flow out of the cells into the mucus, resulting in abnormally thick mucosal secretions. Every person has two CFTR genes, and only one of them needs to be working properly to have normal mucus secretions. Therefore, CF is known as a *recessive* gene, in that both CFTR genes need to have mutations in order for a person to have actual cystic fibrosis disease. People with only one mutated CFTR gene are called carriers and are generally completely asymptomatic, although they will pass this gene on to 50 percent of their biological children.

Many different possible mutations of the CFTR gene exist—over eighteen hundred distinct mutations have already been identified. The most common mutation is the delta F508 deletion, which represents about 70 percent of CFTR gene mutations found on testing. Some mutations are more severe than others in terms of their impairment of the regulation of normal mucosal viscosity. Because of this wide variety of possible mutation combinations, there is a spectrum of cystic fibrosis disease severity. In general, severe impairment of CFTR action results in cystic fibrosis disease and congenital bilateral absence of the vas deferens (CBAVD), whereas mild impairment causes only CBAVD. In between those extremes, there are combinations that can include varying degrees of respiratory impairment combined with CBAVD. Examples include:

Genes	Findings
2 normal CFTR genes	Normal, no problems
1 normal CFTR gene	CFTR carrier, no clinical problems
2 severe CFTR mutations	Cystic fibrosis disease and CBAVD
2 mild CFTR mutations	CBAVD only
1 mild and 1 severe CFTR mutation	Can have CBAVD with or without some degree of respiratory disease

Note that all men with CF have CBAVD, but not all men with CBAVD have CF.

Congenital Bilateral Absence of the Vas Deferens (CBAVD)

The vas deferens carries the sperm from the epididymis to the ejaculatory ducts during ejaculation. Men with two abnormal CFTR genes have abnormal development of the vas deferens and/or ejaculatory ducts, resulting in sperm blockage problems (obstructive azoospermia).

In its most common form, men with CBAVD are missing the entire vas deferens on each side, as well as the body and tail of the epididymis, at least part of the ejaculatory ducts, and sometimes even the seminal vesicles. This results in the complete absence of all fluid from the testicles and seminal vesicles in the ejaculate (but the prostatic fluid can still enter the ejaculate). The clinical presentation of this classic CBAVD scenario includes:

- No palpable vas deferens in the scrotum on either side
- Ejaculate with low volume (under 1.0 cc), acidic pH (under 7.0), and no fructose (since the ejaculate only contains fluid from the prostate gland)
- Ejaculate often looks clear and watery

Variants of CBAVD can occur. Some men are missing only parts of the vas deferens (called "skip lesions") and therefore may have a palpable vas (or part of the vas) in the scrotum on one or both sides. Some men with CBAVD variants may also have an intact ejaculatory duct and therefore have ejaculate with normal alkalinity and fructose, but without sperm. These variants, however, represent a minority of men with CBAVD.

Congenital Unilateral Absence of the Vas Deferens (CUAVD)

CUAVD typically presents with a non-palpable vas deferens on only one side. If the other testicle and genital duct system are intact, semen analysis may be normal. Missing a vas deferens on one side can be associated with CFTR mutation problems about 40 percent of the time. Another cause of CUAVD that is not related to a CFTR gene mutation is a problem with the development of the meso-nephric duct during embryo development. These men are generally missing (on one side) their vas deferens, seminal vesicle, kidney, ureter, and part of their epididymis. CFTR mutation screening and renal ultrasound evaluation are recommended for all men with only one palpable vas deferens.

Congenital Epididymal Obstruction

Some men are born with obstructions in each epididymis. This results in complete azoospermia with a normal semen volume, pH, and fructose. On physical examination, the epididymis on both sides typically feels enlarged or engorged. Congenital epididymal obstruction is associated with a CFTR gene mutation in approxi-mately 45–50 percent of cases, and therefore CFTR screening should be offered to all of these men. Fertility treatment includes microsur-gical reconstruction or sperm extraction combined with IVF/ICSI.

Fertility Treatment of CBAVD

CBAVD and its variants (other than congenital epididymal obstruction) are generally not amenable to surgical reconstruction. Testicular sperm production is usually normal, but FSH blood testing is still recommended in order to make sure sperm produc-tion is still good (see "Hormone Testing in Men" in Chapter 4). If the FSH is normal, then sperm can be extracted from the testicles and used with IVF/ICSI with anticipation of good success rates (see "Management of Obstructive Azoospermia" in Chapter 9). For all men with CFTR mutations, it is important to always screen the female partner for CFTR mutation carrier status. If she is found to also be a carrier of a CFTR gene mutation, then the couple may want to consider preimplantation genetic diagnosis (discussed later in this chapter) to limit the chance of any offspring having cystic fibrosis disease.

Genetic Testing in Men with CBAVD

Men who are suspected of having CBAVD are advised to have genetic testing done to look for mutations of the CFTR gene. CFTR mutation testing is also recommended in men with any other congenital genital duct abnormalities, such as congenital epididymal obstruction or CUAVD (see above). Although there is no gene therapy available at this time, this genetic testing provides important health information for any of the man's siblings and for any children who are conceived, who might be carriers of the same mutations.

If you are considering testing for CFTR mutations, there are several factors to be aware of. One is that CFTR mutations are more common in some ethnic groups than others:

Group	CF carrier rate
Caucasian	1 in 25
Hispanic	1 in 46
African American	1 in 65
Asian	1 in 94

Another is that eighteen hundred different CFTR mutations have been identified, and different specific CFTR mutations are more common in certain ethnic groups. The CF screening test panels used most often have been designed to check for the CFTR gene mutations most frequently found in the Caucasian population, since this group has the highest incidence of the mutation. Therefore, the chance of a false negative result (in which the gene that a person has cannot be identified by a regular screening panel) is higher in non-Caucasian populations.

Group	Rates of false negative screening results for CFTR mutations
Hispanic	1 in 164
Asian	1 in 184
African American	1 in 186
Caucasian	1 in 208

Most commercial CF tests are designed to look for the more severe CFTR mutations that lead to cystic fibrosis. They therefore may not look for some of the more common mild CFTR mutations that cause CBAVD (but not CF). An example of this is the 5T allele of intron 8, which is a common mild CFTR mutation that is not routinely checked in regular CF screening panels.

Which CF screening test should be used? Several different commercially available options exist for CF screening, including a twenty-three-mutation screen, a ninety-seven-mutation screen, and full gene sequencing (note: different labs may modify this a little, and so may have a 100 mutation screen instead of a 97 mutation screen, and these would be essentially equivalent). In general, the standard twenty-three-mutation screen is used in couples without fertility issues who are undergoing a basic screening looking for the most common genes causing CF disease. I prefer to use the ninety-seven-mutation screen (which often includes the 5T allele), as it looks at more of the genes that cause mild CFTR functional loss and can result in CBAVD without CF disease. Full gene sequencing is quite expensive and is not indicated in the majority of patients.

The diagnosis code that can be used is V77.6 (ICD-9). This will change to the ICD-10 code E84 beginning in October 2015.

See Appendix C for the price of CF genetic screening if it is not covered by insurance.

Health Problems Associated with CFTR Mutations

Renal Abnormalities

Because the genital duct and the renal tract have their origins in the same embryonic structure, men with congenital genital duct abnormalities are at a higher risk of having problems with kidney development as well. These problems include having a missing or atrophic (non-functioning) kidney on one side. The incidence of congenital renal problems in men with CBAVD is 10–20 percent, and in men with CUAVD it is 30 percent.

All men with a suspected genital duct development abnormality should have a renal ultrasound to check for the presence of renal anomalies.

Lung Problems

Most men with CBAVD do not have lung problems. However, since the various CFTR gene mutations have different levels of severity, it results in a spectrum of disease. Some CBAVD patients may have some chronic mild lung or sinus problems that can have an impact on their long-term health. CBAVD patients should be asked about a history of such problems as recurrent sinusitis, bronchitis, and pneumonia, and should be followed routinely by their primary care physicians.

Sperm Production

Most men with CBAVD have normal sperm production. However, about 10 percent of these men do have problems making sperm. Therefore, FSH testing is recommended prior to sperm extraction procedures (see "Hormone Testing in Men" in Chapter 4).

Inguinal Hernia

The incidence of inguinal hernias is higher in men with CBAVD (5 percent) than it is in the general population (1.5 percent).

Did CFTR Mutations Provide an Advantage in the Past?

CFTR gene mutations are relatively common in the population because of the survival advantage they gave to people in the distant past. Carrying just one copy of the CFTR gene mutation decreases the amount of fluid loss that a person suffers during diarrhea, and therefore increased their chance of surviving severe diarrheal diseases (such as cholera) in a time before modern medical management. These illnesses were a significant cause of death in the past, and continue to be in some countries.

Kallmann Syndrome

Kallmann syndrome (KS) is a genetic abnormality that usually involves a mutation of the KAL-1 gene. Typically only men are clinically affected, because it is an X-linked condition and they have just one X chromosome; women are usually just carriers, because they have two X chromosomes, and if the other X chromosome is normal, they do not develop symptoms. Men with KS have no GnRH secretion from the hypothalamus area of the brain, which in turn leads to no FSH and LH production by the anterior pituitary gland. Men with KS are therefore usually azoospermic, with low FSH, LH, and testosterone levels. Men with KS are most often diagnosed as teenagers, when they undergo an evaluation because of delayed onset of puberty.

Kallmann syndrome can be associated with other abnormalities as well, including:

- Facial/cranial asymmetry
- Renal abnormalities or failure to develop
- Cryptorchidism

- Cleft palate

- Gynecomastia

- Color blindness

- Cerebellar dysfunction

- Congenital deafness

- Neurologic abnormalities

A definitive diagnosis of KS can be difficult, as it is not detected by normal karyotype testing. Specific testing for the KAL-1 gene on the X chromosome can be performed, and can provide a diagnosis if the entire gene is absent. However, multiple genes on several different chromosomes may also play a role in the development of Kallmann syndrome, and the absence of these genes (or only small abnormalities of the KAL-1 gene) may not be detected with KAL-1 gene testing. Genetic counselors should be involved in making the decision about testing for KS.

The primary fertility issue in men with Kallmann syndrome is a lack of gonadotropins (FSH and LH). These men typically respond well to LH and FSH replacement therapy. Treatment is generally started with HCG. If sperm have not returned after six months of therapy, then FSH is added. On this regimen, sperm can be expected to return in 90 percent of men with KS. Despite the fact that in about 70 percent of these men sperm counts do not reach normal levels, most are able to conceive naturally or with use of low-tech treatments such as IUI. Genetic counseling is recommended for couples prior to undergoing fertility treatments using the man's sperm.

Other Genetic Abnormalities

46 XX Syndrome

Men with a 46 XX karyotype have had part of the Y chromosome (called the sex-determining region Y gene, or SRY gene) translocated to the X chromosome. The SRY gene is responsible for the development of male anatomy and appearance. However, the rest of the genes on the Y chromosome that are responsible for sperm production (including the AZF region) are missing. Men with 46 XX are therefore completely azoospermic, and they typically have small, firm testicles with high FSH and low testosterone levels. Attempted sperm extractions with methods such as mTESE will not be successful in finding sperm, since the entire AZF region of the chromosome is missing. For these men, adoption, donor sperm, or donor embryos are the only options for having children.

47 XYY Syndrome

The 47 XYY karyotype occurs in approximately one in a thousand live male births. It is associated with increased height, but past theories of an association with aggressive and antisocial behavior have been mostly dismissed. Some men with 47 XYY are fertile, but there are high rates of severe oligospermia and azoospermia in this population. Lab values typically show normal testosterone and LH levels but high FSH levels. Most of the sperm produced by these men are genetically normal, but genetic counseling and preimplantation genetic diagnosis (PGD) are recommended if the couple wishes to decrease the chance of passing on the same genetic abnormality to offspring.

Preimplantation Genetic Diagnosis (PGD) and Preimplantation Genetic Screening (PGS)

Preimplantation Genetic Diagnosis (PGD)

PGD is a technique that can be used to genetically evaluate embryos during an IVF cycle before these embryos have been transferred into the woman's uterus. Traditionally, PGD has been used in conjunction with IVF to see if a developing embryo in the lab is harboring certain single-gene abnormalities. PGD was first introduced in 1990 and has primarily been used in couples with known heritable genetic problems. Common diseases for which PGD is used include:

- Sickle cell anemia
- Cystic fibrosis
- Beta thalassemia
- Myotonic dystrophy type I
- Huntington's disease
- Familial adenomatous polyposis

Traditionally with PGD, once the embryo reached the eight-cell stage on day 3 (when it is called a blastomere), one cell would be removed and sent for genetic evaluation. The results of the genetic testing would be available by day 5, when blastocyst transfer of those embryos that did not harbor the genetic abnormalities in question would be done. PGD has several downsides:

- There is some evidence that embryo biopsy may modestly decrease IVF success rates
- The woman must generate a sufficient number of eggs to have enough day-3 embryos to biopsy; she also must have enough progressing day-5 embryos to transfer, which may be difficult in women with decreased ovulatory reserve.

- Embryo mosaicism (in which different cells in the same embryo have different genetic makeups) can decrease the accuracy of finding an abnormality when only one cell is tested.

To address the problem of embryo mosaicism, multicellular biopsies (called trophoectoderm biopsies) are now often performed on the day-5 or day-6 embryo (blastocyst). However, a trade-off is that the embryos must then be frozen (vitrified) while waiting for the results of the genetic testing, and some experts think this embryo cryopreservation can modestly decrease IVF success rates, although not all specialists agree.

Generally, PGD is thought to be about 90 percent accurate. Due to the 10 percent error rate, fetal testing such as chorionic villus sampling (done at 10–14 weeks) or amniocentesis (at 15–22 weeks) is also recommended for prenatal diagnosis.

The cost of PGD is usually in the range of an extra $3,000 to $6,000 and is typically not covered by insurance, even if a couple has insurance coverage for IVF.

Gender Balancing

Gender balancing involves performing PGD for the primary purpose of choosing the sex of a child. Most IVF laboratories do not routinely offer gender balancing.

Preimplantation Genetic Screening (PGS)

More recently, the techniques of PGD have been used in couples to attempt to maximize their chances of success with IVF. PGS screens for genetic abnormalities in all twenty-three chromosome pairs, as opposed to PGD, which just looks for a single genetic defect that one of the parents is known to carry. Some centers now offer PGS for couples who have experienced recurrent IVF implantation failure or recurrent pregnancy loss, or in which the woman is older.

PGS has an obvious appeal for couples who have had several failed IVF cycles for unknown reasons, and some studies have shown improvements in fertility outcomes with its use. However, other studies have shown no benefit with the use of PGS, with some even showing decreased pregnancy rates, presumably due to the negative impact of embryo biopsy and the need to often freeze the embryo prior to transfer. The American Society of Reproductive Medicine maintains that current studies do not support the use of PGS to improve pregnancy rates or decrease miscarriage rates with IVF, though some fertility experts disagree and feel that it can play an important role in increasing success rates.

11

Advanced Sperm Testing

This chapter is for couples who have suspected functional sperm problems that go beyond the standard semen parameters of density, motility, and morphology. At this point in time, advanced sperm testing is not indicated in most couples who are having trouble conceiving. The most common candidates for advanced sperm testing are couples who have failed multiple cycles of IVF for unknown reasons, especially in the presence of poor embryo progression and/or poor embryo quality (see below). Some advanced sperm tests, such as DNA fragmentation index, can also be performed for couples with unexplained recurrent pregnancy loss.

A wide array of advanced sperm tests are currently under evaluation by the scientific community. Although many potentially promising tests have been discovered, none has yet proven to be the game-changing breakthrough that everyone is looking for. When one of these new tests is developed, it tends to follow a particular pattern in which the initial research studies on a small number of patients show a significant positive correlation between the sperm test results and fertility outcomes. The clinical fertility community gets excited that a breakthrough in sperm testing has been found that will change the treatment options for couples with recurrent IVF failures. However, subsequent larger-scale studies by other institutions often find that these tests are not quite as clinically useful as first anticipated, and the search goes on.

The holy grail of advanced sperm testing is a test that will have the ability to not only determine which patients have high levels of functional sperm impairment but also determine which individual sperm have good fertility potential and isolate them for use in IVF/ICSI. Unfortunately, no test to date can do all this. However, several tests have shown themselves to be potentially clinically useful:

- DNA fragmentation index (DFI)
- Intracytoplasmic morphologically selected sperm injection (IMSI)
- Hyaluronan binding assay (HBA)
- Birefringence testing of sperm heads using polarized light
- Raman spectroscopy
- Membrane-based electrophoresis
- Microfluidic testing
- Magnetic activated cell sorting (MACS)

Later sections in this chapter will review a few of these tests in further detail, including the sperm DNA fragmentation testing, IMSI, and HBA. This does not mean that these are necessarily the best of the above-listed tests, only that these three seem to have the most published scientific data associated with them to date.

Recurrent IVF Failure

There can be several possible reasons for a couple to fail multiple cycles of IVF, including functional sperm problems, functional egg problems, a combination of sperm and egg problems, and plain bad luck with earlier cycles.

In the absence of a good explanation for multiple IVF failures, further advanced testing of the couple is an option, to see if there are any reversible factors that may indicate ways to increase the chances of success with subsequent IVF cycles. Since a woman's eggs are inaccessible to direct testing, interest has focused on the testing of sperm to look for any functional abnormalities that may be contributing to a couple's infertility problems. Sperm functional contributions are especially suspect when the problem during the IVF cycle seems to be poor embryo progression or quality, since sperm quality usually has the greatest impact on IVF/ICSI outcomes during embryo development. In IVF, the first phase of sperm/egg interaction is fertilization, where the sperm and egg fuse to form an embryo. Normal fertilization rates are generally thought to be in the 70–75 percent range. Fertilization is primarily under the control of the egg's genetic material, although the sperm does make a few minor contributions. Therefore, problems with egg fertilization, such as poor fertilization rates, are usually thought to be more related to either egg issues or simple bad luck.

Following fertilization, the embryo begins to rapidly divide in a process called embryo development. The male genetic material seems to play a much more important role in embryo development starting at the eight-cell stage. Therefore, if a couple has had several failed cycles of IVF, the timing of when problems appeared can offer clues about whether sperm DNA factors may be playing a role. If poor fertilization (that is, low fertilization rates) is the primary problem, then it is less likely that the sperm DNA is a contributing factor, although this cannot be concluded with 100 percent certainty. If, however, fertilization rates have been good but embryo progression or quality has been the primary problem, this suggests that poor sperm DNA quality may be playing a role.

Sperm DNA Fragmentation Testing

When a sperm successfully enters an egg, the twenty-three chromosomes of its DNA must fuse with the egg's twenty-three chromosomes in order to form the full forty-six chromosomes of the resulting embryo. As described earlier, the male's DNA contribution generally starts to play a role after fertilization has occurred, and therefore abnormalities in sperm DNA typically play a larger role in subsequent embryo development.

Nuclear chromatin is the material combination of DNA, RNA, and proteins in the nucleus of cells. Most of the body's cells have robust mechanisms to defend against damage to the cell's DNA, as well as the ability to repair some types of damage that do occur. Unfortunately, the sperm cell has a very different structure compared to most other cell types in the body, because it needs to be compact, mobile, and strong enough to swim long distances and successfully interact with an awaiting egg. Because it has a unique membrane structure and a very limited supply of antioxidants, sperm are especially susceptible to damage by reactive oxygen species. In addition, sperm have only minimal ability to repair any DNA damage that they might sustain.

Sperm DNA integrity can be evaluated by one of three methods:

- DNA fragmentation index (DFI; also called SCSA and SDFA)
- TUNEL (terminal deoxynucleotidyl transferase dUTP nick end labeling)
- Comet assay (single cell gel electrophoresis)

All three of these testing methods are reliable, and their findings correlate fairly well with each other. The one most commonly used commercially is DFI testing. At this time, the TUNEL and comet assays are more frequently used in research at large research institutions, which perform the testing in their own labs. The TUNEL assay does have the advantage of being able to test the DNA fragmentation index of very small numbers of sperm, including those extracted from the testicle (as opposed to DFI testing, in which a sperm density of at least 1 million per cc is generally required).

While sperm DNA testing offers another useful way to examine the ability of sperm to interact successfully with an egg that goes beyond the standard semen parameters of density, motility, and morphology, at this point in time sperm genetic testing can only tell us what percentage of sperm have normal DNA versus abnormal DNA. No sperm DNA test can currently identify specifically which sperm have normal DNA and then select those exact sperm with intact DNA to be used with IVF/ICSI.

Sperm DNA testing is offered by several different companies. See Appendix C.

DNA Fragmentation Index (DFI)

The most widespread, commercially available assay for assessing sperm DNA integrity is DFI testing. Commercially, DFI testing can be found under such names as SDFA (sperm DNA fragmentation assay) and SCSA (sperm chromatin structure assay).

DFI testing is an indirect assay that measures the ability of sperm chromatin to resist DNA denaturation after exposure to stress, such as a mild acid. In this test, around five thousand sperm are evaluated by a process called flow cytometry, and results are given as a percentage of sperm cells with fragmented DNA.

Normal DFI is under 30 percent (that is, less than 30 percent of sperm exhibit fragmentation when exposed to stress). Often labs will define a borderline DFI result range of 20–30 percent, but most guidelines consider 30 percent to be the actual normal cutoff.

Studies have shown that healthy fertile males typically have a DFI of around 20 percent.

Elevated levels of DFI are found in about 10 percent of normal fertile men versus 20–30 percent of infertile men. Studies have found that about 8 percent of infertile men who have normal standard semen parameters have an abnormally high DFI on testing. DFI levels are not necessarily correlated with semen parameters and have only a weak correlation with strict morphology findings.

Causes of increased sperm DFI include:

- Oxidative stress (the most common cause), such as that associated with pyospermia
- Tobacco use
- Excessive heat exposure (for example, using a laptop computer on the lap, or using a hot tub)
- Obesity
- Chemotherapy or radiation therapy
- Air pollution exposure
- Varicoceles
- Aging (DFI is about 13 percent in men between twenty and twenty-nine years old, versus about 50 percent in men between sixty and eighty)
- Prolonged sexual abstinence
- Spinal cord injury
- SSRI use (healthy volunteers taking paroxetine [Paxil] had an average increase in sperm DFI from 14 percent to 30 percent after four weeks of use, with no change in standard semen parameters)

Impact of DFI on Fertility Outcomes

The impact of a high DFI on fertility varies significantly between couples. One reason for this is that a woman's egg is able to repair some degree of sperm DNA damage, and this amount of repair varies among individuals—for example, eggs from younger women may have more repair capacity.

Abnormal DFI has been associated with poorer outcomes for natural intercourse, IUI, standard IVF, and IVF/ICSI.

- Natural intercourse: a DFI over 30 percent is associated with a 7-fold decrease in the rate of natural conception
- Intrauterine insemination: a DFI over 30 percent is associated with a 7.3-fold decrease in pregnancy rate
- Standard IVF: a DFI over 30 percent is associated with a 2-fold decrease in pregnancy rate
- IVF/ICSI: a DFI over 30 percent is associated with a 1.5-fold decrease in pregnancy rate (although some experts think that DFI has a minimal impact if ICSI is used)

Sperm DNA testing is still relatively new, and the above findings need to be verified by additional large, controlled studies. Currently the American Society of Reproductive Medicine does not recommend sperm DFI testing for routine male fertility evaluations. However, there is emerging compelling evidence that DFI testing can play a useful role in several specific clinical situations: recurrent unexplained pregnancy loss, recurrent unexplained IVF failure, and couples in which the man's semen analysis is normal but who still have unexplained persistent infertility.

Couples with otherwise normal semen parameters who are not having success with timed intercourse or intrauterine insemination can have sperm DFI testing to help them decide if moving straight to IVF/ICSI would be beneficial (if a highly abnormal DFI is found) versus trying longer with the low-tech treatments (if the DFI is normal). Some clinicians also use sperm DNA testing to assess the integrity of sperm DNA in various at-risk populations, such as post-chemotherapy patients or older men, although no official guidelines have yet been established.

Treatment of Elevated Sperm DFI

Three main approaches are usually undertaken to reduce DFI fragmentation levels in men with abnormal testing, including antioxidant therapy, treatment of reversible risk factors, and maximizing the freshness of the sperm specimen.

Antioxidant therapy (see "General Recommendations for All Men Trying to Conceive," in Chapter 5) can decrease sperm DFI by protecting DNA from damaging free radicals.

Reversible risk factors known to increase sperm DFI can be managed, including:

- Stopping tobacco use
- Weight loss in obese patients
- Avoidance of excessive heat (hot tubs, saunas, etc.)
- Treatment of clinically significant varicoceles (see "Varicoceles" in Chapter 6)
- Change from a SSRI antidepressant to another type of anti-depressant medication (such as Wellbutrin) that may have less impact on sperm ductal transport (this should be done under the care of the patient's primary care provider or psychiatrist)

Most sperm DNA fragmentation occurs within the epididymis and genital duct system; less occurs in the testicles. Therefore, getting the freshest sperm possible can decrease the sperm DFI in some men. I generally have men with sperm DFI problems who have an upcoming sperm DFI test or IVF cycle ejaculate daily for one week, and then abstain for one day prior to collecting their semen specimen. Studies have shown that in men with an elevated DFI, daily ejaculations for a week can potentially decrease DFI readings by over 40 percent.

Some men with unexplained IVF failure or pregnancy loss cannot decrease their DFI to the normal range despite all of the above interventions. Several small studies have shown that in these circumstances, sperm surgically taken directly from the testicle typically have lower DFI scores than ejaculated sperm (DFI 24–40 percent with ejaculated sperm vs. 5–13 percent with testicular sperm). These extracted sperm can then be used for IVF/ICSI. Small studies have found higher pregnancy rates using these fresh extracted sperm when compared with cycles that used the ejaculated sperm. It is controversial as to whether sperm freezing significantly increases sperm DFI in men with abnormal fragmentation levels to begin with. In men with normal fertility, any mild increase in DFI associated with freezing likely has little clinical impact. However, to optimize sperm quality, I prefer to use fresh sperm extractions for men with persistently elevated DFI levels and recurrent IVF failure.

High DNA Stainability (HDS)

Some sperm DNA tests include an HDS evaluation, which measures the percentage of sperm cells with immature chromatin. Elevated HDS levels indicate the presence of higher levels of immature sperm. In men with sperm production problems, increased numbers of immature sperm are often present on standard semen analysis testing (see "White Blood Cells or Round Cells" in Chapter 3). The presence of immature sperm cells can potentially increase oxidative stress on the sperm. In healthy, fertile men, average HDS is about 6 percent, though up to 15 percent is still considered normal.

Elevated HDS readings have been associated with longer times to pregnancy with IUI and IVF in some studies. However, at this point in time, I do not think the clinical data supporting HDS testing are particularly compelling.

Intracytoplasmic Morphologically Selected Sperm Injection (IMSI)

IMSI is an intervention that can be performed at the time of IVF/ICSI and is used to select the best-quality sperm to be injected into each egg. This technique (motile sperm organelle morphology examination, or MSOME) is based upon evaluating sperm at very high magnifications using a specially designed microscope. Standard ICSI evaluations of sperm generally take place at 300–400× magnification, while IMSI evaluates sperm at magnifications of up to 6,000×. This allows a more thorough assessment of sperm cell structure, including evaluation for specific structures such as vacuoles within the sperm heads.

Studies have shown that approximately 65 percent of sperm that were selected under standard 300–400× magnification as good candidates for use with ICSI in fact showed abnormalities of sperm structure when evaluated at 6,000× magnification with IMSI. Various studies have found that sperm assessed as having normal shape under IMSI evaluation had lower levels of genetic aneuploidy (abnormal number of chromosomes) and lower levels of DNA fragmentation. Some studies have shown improved embryo quality (after day 3), increased pregnancy rates, improved embryo implantation rates, and decreased miscarriage rates when IMSI-selected sperm are used. Improved pregnancy rates have also been found when IMSI is used in couples who have failed multiple cycles of standard IVF/ICSI.

Despite the promising findings of these studies, other studies have shown no improvement in fertility outcomes with IMSI. A 2013 Cochrane Review looking at all the available good-quality studies did not find compelling evidence of improvements in fertility outcomes or decreases in miscarriage rates with the use of IMSI, and concluded that further trials are necessary before IMSI can be recommended in clinical practice. Other downsides to IMSI are that it is a very time-consuming process and that it is not widely available in the United States at this time.

The cost of IMSI is going to be different for each institution, and is also likely going to vary depending upon the number of eggs that are retrieved for IVF (as more eggs means that more better-quality sperm need to be identified to inject into each egg). In general the cost of IMSI at a facility will likely range between $2,500 and $4,000.

My overall impression is that IMSI has the potential to be of help to couples who have failed multiple cycles of IVF/ICSI due to poor embryo quality or progression and are trying to optimize their chances of success for a subsequent cycle. I hope that future clinical data will support the role of IMSI for couples with recurrent unexplained IVF failures, and that this technology will become more available in the United States at a reduced cost.

Hyaluronan Binding Assay (HBA)

The human egg is surrounded by a layer called the cumulus oophorus complex, which is primarily made up of a substance called hyaluronic acid. This layer acts as an efficient sperm selection barrier, since only mature, normally functioning sperm are generally allowed to pass through and initiate fertilization. Sperm that are able to bind to hyaluronic acid have been shown in some studies to have lower levels of sperm DNA fragmentation, resulting in better embryo quality and development.

Testing of sperm binding to hyaluronic acid has been used in two ways:

- *Hyaluronan binding assay (HBA).* This simple, inexpensive test looks at the percentage of sperm that will successfully bind to hyaluronic acid. Normal levels have been reported to range from 60 percent to 80 percent or higher. Some labs have used this test in couples who need IVF, but it remains unclear whether standard IVF or IVF/ICSI should be used. If the HBA shows abnormally low binding, then that patient's sperm may have trouble with normal egg/sperm interactions, and adding ICSI may improve the couple's outcomes. The average cost of HBA is $50.

- *PICSI (physiologic ICSI).* This involves exposing sperm to a sheet of hyaluronic acid, and then choosing sperm for ICSI from those that have successfully been bound after five to ten minutes of incubation. The thinking is that these bound sperm are potentially healthier. Some studies have shown that using these sperm results in improvements in embryo quality and implantation rates, with a trend toward improved fertilization and pregnancy rates with PICSI (as opposed to standard ICSI). However, other studies have not shown improvements in fertility outcomes using PICSI. A potential criticism is that PICSI may be choosing sperm with lower overall motility, since the poorly motile are easily bound, while extremely motile sperm may break free and so not be identified for use with ICSI. The cost of PICSI is going to vary between labs. The PICSI dishes themselves are produced by Origio and are not particularly expensive, but there is lab time involved with using them and selecting out the bound sperm. My estimation of a general cost for PICSI based upon other lab related activities would be about $500 to $1,000.

I think HBA testing may provide some useful information about men who might benefit from IVF/ICSI as opposed to standard IVF. PICSI might also be of benefit in men with recurrent IVF/ICSI failure of unknown cause, although more studies are needed to prove definitive improvements in pregnancy and live birth rates.

Oxidative Stress Adduct Test

Specialized testing is available that can directly measure the degree of oxidative damage affecting a man's sperm. For the oxidative stress adduct (OSA) test, a normal result is under 3.8, a borderline result is between 3.8 and 4.4, and an abnormal result is over 4.4.

OSA testing is available from Reprosource (www.reprosource.com) and is part of their Advanced Semen Report, which also includes DNA fragmentation index testing. The cost of the Advanced Semen Report is $175 if insurance does not cover the test. The shipping and handling cost for a home collection of the specimen is $75, but this may be less if the sample is collected at a fertility center that performs routine semen analysis.

I do not typically order OSA testing for male fertility patients, as I routinely place almost all of these men on an inexpensive, over-the-counter regimen of antioxidants and work on reducing oxidative stress risk factors (such as smoking). However, in some circumstances OSA testing may be useful. An example would be a man with persistent pyospermia that is resistant to treatment. OSA testing can potentially provide information about whether the sperm are still experiencing oxidative stress despite antioxidant therapy, in which case sperm wash and IUI may be helpful.

See "Elevated White Blood Cells (Pyospermia)" in Chapter 6 for more information on the management of pyospermia, which is a common source of oxidative stress.

Post-Coital Testing

Post-coital testing (PCT) involves evaluating the woman's cervical mucus microscopically for the presence of sperm following intercourse. The test must be performed in the peri-ovulatory period (when the cervical mucus is most receptive to sperm) and approximately two to eight hours after intercourse. A normal test result is defined as more than 10 sperm per high power field (hpf) under the microscope.

PCT is not commonly performed, but it may be useful when there is concern regarding sperm delivery to the cervical mucus. Potential reasons for ordering PCT testing include:

- Hyperviscous semen
- Unexplained infertility
- Low volume ejaculate with normal sperm count
- Evaluating the fertility potential of men who are not able to produce a specimen either with masturbation or with a special collection condom
- Concerns about cervical problems
- Proximal hypospadias when there are concerns that sperm are not being deposited near the cervix

Rarely Used Sperm Tests

Other fertility testing methods that are not used much anymore include several tests to evaluate the sperm/egg interactions needed for normal egg fertilization. In the pre-ICSI era, this was important information, as only standard IVF was available, in which about 100,000 sperm were mixed with each egg in a sterile laboratory dish, so the sperm and egg had to interact together normally. These interactions include such necessary steps as capacitation (biochemical changes within the sperm when it enters into the female reproductive tract that make it able to fertilize an egg) and acrosome reaction (when the sperm binds to the zona pellucida surrounding the egg, it initiates the acrosome reaction within the sperm, causing a release of enzymes from the acrosome cap, which allows the sperm to penetrate the egg and initiate fertilization).

The ability to perform intra-cytoplasmic sperm injection (ICSI), in which a single sperm is injected directly into each egg, has made the determination of egg-sperm interactions less important. Poor fertilization rates with standard IVF are now routinely managed with IVF/ICSI, thereby bypassing the need for cumbersome egg/sperm interaction testing. These tests are briefly described for historical purposes only, as they are only rarely used now. These outdated tests include:

- Acrosome reaction testing, designed to see if the sperm has a normal release of acrosomal enzymes. Used in the past for men with profound abnormalities of sperm heads and in couples with standard IVF failure. Downsides included no absolute cutoffs for normal values and limited lab availability.

- Sperm penetration assay, which tests the ability of sperm to penetrate an egg to initiate fertilization. Sperm are mixed in the lab with hamster ova and evaluated for their ability to penetrate the egg.

- Sperm zona binding, which tests the ability of the sperm to attach to the zona pellucida (outer covering of the egg).

12

Vasectomy Reversal

Vasectomy is a very common form of birth control used in the United States. Approximately 5 percent of men who have had a vasectomy subsequently change their minds, however, and want to have more children in the future. The good news is that there are several options with high rates of success that men can pursue to have more children who are biologically related to them.

When a man has undergone a vasectomy for contraception, the testicles continue to make sperm, but these sperm are reabsorbed by the body, since they are blocked and have nowhere to go. Any man considering have children following a previous vasectomy should have testing to make sure that he has continued good sperm production, since this is important for good fertility outcomes. FSH blood testing is more than 90 percent accurate in predicting that sperm production is still good (see "Hormone Testing in Men" in Chapter 4 for more information on FSH testing). As long as sperm production is still reasonable, then post-vasectomy men who wish to have children who are biologically related to them have two options: sperm extraction combined with IVF/ICSI, or microscopic vasectomy reversal.

Sperm Extraction Procedure

If sperm production is still good, then a sperm extraction procedure is generally highly successful in terms of obtaining enough sperm for use in fertility procedures; the success rate is 90 to 95 percent. "Management of Obstructive Azoospermia" in Chapter 9 reviews in detail the different types of sperm extraction procedures. In Ohio, the total cost for a sperm extraction procedure is generally around $3,000 ($1,000 for the procedure, $1,000 for the facility fee and anesthesia, and $1,000 for the fertility lab fee to process, freeze, and store the sperm.

The key point to note with a sperm extraction is that the sperm cannot be used for intrauterine insemination, as extracted sperm are not mature enough to swim up the fallopian tubes and fertilize an egg naturally. The sperm need to be used in conjunction with IVF/ICSI, in which a single sperm is injected into each retrieved egg at the fertility laboratory (see Appendix D for more detailed information on IVF/ICSI). The cost for a cycle of IVF in Ohio is generally around $12,000–$13,000.

If you are interested in this route, then the first step is generally for the female partner to see an IVF doctor to make sure that she is a good candidate for IVF. The IVF doctor usually works with a local urologist to perform the sperm extraction procedure. Unlike vasectomy reversals, most men do not need to travel to find an expert in sperm extraction, as this is a much less technically demanding procedure. As mentioned before, FSH testing on the man is recommended to make sure that his sperm production is still good prior to proceeding.

Microscopic Vasectomy Reversal

A microscopic vasectomy reversal is the second option to have a biologically related child following a previous vasectomy. The advantages of a vasectomy reversal include the fact that the procedure is limited to only the male (as opposed to the extraction/IVF route, in which both partners need to have invasive procedures), it allows for natural conception to occur, and it allows the couple to try for more than one child without the need for additional procedures.

The goal of a vasectomy reversal is to surgically reestablish the flow of sperm from the testicles to the urethra through the vas deferens. The vas is quite small, with an outer diameter of 2–4 mm (in comparison, a standard #2 pencil has an outer diameter of 6–7 mm). The walls of the vas deferens are thick and muscular, so the lumen, the inside channel where the sperm travel, is significantly smaller yet, with a diameter of only 0.3–0.5 mm (in comparison, the thickness of a standard sheet of copy paper is 0.1 mm). The use of precise surgical technique is essential to prevent scar tissue from blocking the channel again after a reversal. If the surgeon is performing a careful, two-layered microsurgical reanastomosis, the reversal procedure generally takes approximately two and a half to three hours of actual operating time.

There are two ways in which a vasectomy reversal can be performed. One option is to attach one end of the vas deferens to the other, which is called a vasovasostomy (or vas-to-vas connection). The scarred, blocked areas where the vas deferens had been cut, tied, or cauterized during the original vasectomy are removed during the reversal procedure, so fresh, healthy tissue is brought together for optimal healing.

The other option is to connect the vas deferens to the epididymis, a procedure that is called a vasoepididymostomy (or vas-to-epididymis connection). The epididymis is the structure that wraps around the side of the testicle; it is where sperm maturation takes place. The epididymal tubules are smaller than the vas deferens, and therefore they can be blocked off with even very small amounts of scar tissue. Therefore, a vas-to-vas connection has a higher chance of success, and is always performed if possible.

It cannot be known until the reversal procedure is under way whether a vas-to-vas or vas-to-epididymis connection will be needed. The decision is made by the surgeon, who examines the fluid that comes from the end of the vas deferens going toward the testicle when it is opened. A drop of this fluid is placed on a glass slide and examined under a tabletop microscope in the operating room; the vasal fluid is checked individually on each side. Favorable fluid (clear or thin and milky in appearance, sperm or sperm parts present) indicates that the path flowing from the testicle to the site of the prior vasectomy is not blocked and a vas-to-vas connection can be performed. However, if thick, creamy fluid without sperm is found, it indicates that one of the delicate epididymal tubules has previously ruptured under the back pressure of the blocked sperm. An epididymal rupture typically does not cause any symptoms (such as pain), but it does obstruct the transport of sperm beyond the rupture site. When this occurs, a vas-to-epididymis connection is needed in order to bypass the area of epididymal blockage, and the vas is attached to the epididymis at a point where sperm are found above the rupture site. The chance of needing a vas-to-epididymis connection is greater if it has been longer since the vasectomy was performed. If the surgeon does not know how to perform a vas-to-epididymis connection when necessary, then the reversal procedure almost certainly will not be successful on the side that requires it.

Success Rates

The chances for sperm returning in good numbers (when performed by a fellowship-trained microsurgical specialist) depends on the type of connections that were needed at the time of the reversal:

- Vas-to-vas on both sides: 90–95 percent
- Vas-to-vas on one side and vas-to-epididymis on the other: 75–80 percent
- Vas-to-epididymis on both sides: 55–60 percent

You may see higher success rates posted on some websites. There are two things to keep in mind when assessing quoted success rates. The first is that you have to trust that the surgeon is posting true numbers, as there is no independent fact-checking system. The numbers listed above match closely with the peer-reviewed scientific studies, with verifiable sources, that fellowship-trained specialists have published over the years in scientific journals.

The second point to consider is what a particular surgeon is defining as "success." The numbers listed above refer to the chances of a man who has had a reversal getting back to relatively normal numbers of swimming sperm, where natural conception would be a likely event. Some websites will list success rates of 98 percent or higher, but when you look into the description of "success" (if there is one), it may be defined as *any* number of sperm returning to the ejaculate. If only a handful of sperm are present following a reversal, the doctor may count this as a statistical "success," but it certainly would not be one in terms of a couple's chances of conception.

Choosing a Vasectomy Reversal Specialist

As described above, the first step for a man considering a vasectomy reversal is to have an FSH blood test done, to make sure that his sperm production is still good. Once it has been determined that sperm production is still good, the next step is to identify the physician with whom you would like to have the procedure performed. The initial reaction of some men is to go back to the urologist who did their initial vasectomy, especially if they had a good experience with that doctor. The problem with this approach is that although almost all urologists receive adequate training and experience in performing standard vasectomies, very few of them learn the latest, most specialized microsurgical techniques for vasectomy reversals.

Choosing your vasectomy reversal surgeon is probably the single most important factor contributing to successful outcomes. Unfortunately, some men face a difficult decision when trying to figure out whom they should choose to perform their reversal. While almost all doctors who offer the vasectomy reversal procedure describe themselves as "microsurgical experts," only a small percentage of them have truly undergone advanced fertility microsurgical training. This section is designed to help you identify which doctors are true specialists in male fertility microsurgery.

There are basically three types of doctors who offer vasectomy reversal procedures:

- *Non-urologists.* These doctors are the "bargain" vasectomy reversal doctors who market themselves extensively on the Internet. They are almost never urologists, but typically doctors who trained in other fields, such as orthopedics or general surgery. Without even looking into their background training, you can almost always identify these non-urologists by their offer of a very cheap reversal ($3,000 or less) under local anesthesia in their office. I strongly urge you to be wary of any non-urologists offering cheap reversals under local anesthesia, regardless of how persuasive their websites may appear.

- *General urologists.* These doctors have completed basic urologic training and are very proficient at treating general urologic issues, such as kidney stones and prostate problems. General urologists have learned the skills to allow them to safely operate within the scrotum. However, the teaching of advanced microsurgical skills is typically quite limited during general urologic training, with very few learning the latest reversal techniques. Thus, while they are certainly more likely to be qualified to perform a vasectomy reversal than a non-urologist, without additional focused training most general urologists are still not optimally trained to provide the most effective procedure possible.

- *Fellowship-trained microsurgical specialists.* These doctors are board-certified urologists who have completed further advanced fellowship training in order to master the latest, most effective microsurgical vasectomy reversal techniques. Less than 1–2 percent of urologists choose to complete a full one-to-two-year fellowship training program in microsurgery, so these specialists are rather few and far between. Nevertheless, they are worth seeking out in order to have the best odds for a successful vasectomy reversal. Additionally, they have had focused, formal training in male fertility issues, and their input can be invaluable in helping to optimize fertility potential following a reversal.

Some couples just look for the cheapest procedure possible, or are in the unfortunate circumstance of absolutely not being able to afford anything more than $3,000 (even with available financing options). If price is the only consideration, then such couples may be content with seeing a "bargain" non-urologist for a quick (one- to one-and-a-half-hour) reversal procedure under local anesthesia. A certain percentage of these cheap, quick reversal procedures will be successful, and a particular couple just might get lucky.

However, for couples who have the resources, the services of a true fertility microsurgical expert provide their best chance of having a successful reversal. A couple's first attempt at a reversal always offers the greatest chance of success, as any subsequent attempts have more associated scar tissue as well as an increased risk of needing a potentially less successful vas-to-epididymis connection. This is to say that if a first attempt at reversal fails, a second attempt may be possible, but it almost certainly will be more challenging, and success rates will be lower than can be expected for a first try.

The good news is that there is an easy way to identify a true microsurgical expert: simply ask the doctor (or the doctor's staff) if he or she is a board-certified urologist who has completed a one-to-two-year fellowship in male fertility and microsurgery. (The difference between a one-year fellowship and a two-year fellowship is not significant clinically, as the extra fellowship year is generally spent doing research in a lab.) Do not be afraid to ask this very important question!

A more detailed explanation of how to identify true microsurgical experts can be found by visiting my website at www.vasectomy-reversal-expert.com.

Four Questions You Should Ask Any Vasectomy Reversal Surgeon

1. *Is the doctor a urologist?* If yes, then at a minimum you are assured that the surgeon has had four to five years of training in scrotal surgery and can offer you as safe a procedure as possible. The same could not be said of a non-urologist offering to do scrotal surgery (although, unfortunately, such doctors do exist). You would not seek out a urologist to treat a fractured arm, so why would you travel to another state to have an orthopedic surgeon perform complex urologic mi-

crosurgery? At a bare minimum, make sure that you are seeing a urologist. Ask directly if it is not apparent.

2. *Will the actual operating time be at least two to two and a half
   hours?* This does not include the time you will be at the office or surgery center or in the recovery area, but only how
   long the surgeon will be actively performing the procedure.
   The leading fellowship-trained experts usually require several hours to perform the latest, most effective techniques. If
   your procedure is going to last only an hour to an hour and
   a half, then it is highly unlikely that the most advanced (and
   successful) surgical techniques are being used. It just does
   not make logical sense that a precise surgery of this delicate
   nature can be performed in half the time by a surgeon with
   less training, so be cautious if that is what is offered.

3. *Does the surgeon know how to perform an expert vas-to-
   epididymis connection if unfavorable vasal fluid is found at the
   time of the reversal?* Unfavorable fluid can be found regardless of how long it has been since a vasectomy was
   performed, so fluid should be checked in all men during
   their operation. If unfavorable fluid is found at the time of a
   reversal and the surgeon does not know how to perform a
   vas-to-epididymis connection, then the reversal will almost
   invariably be unsuccessful on that side. It is therefore critical
   that your surgeon be prepared to check the vasal fluid and
   perform a vas-to-epididymis connection if necessary.

4. *Has the urologist completed a one-to-two-year fellowship in male
   infertility and microsurgery?* If you ask only one question, this
   should be the one, because if you are working with a fellowship-trained microsurgical specialist, then the answer to all
   three questions listed above will almost invariably be yes.
   Having completed a fellowship in fertility microsurgery is

the only sure sign that the surgeon with whom you are working has invested the time and energy needed to become a true microsurgical reversal expert. I emphasize this so strongly because there are so many physicians offering reversals without having expert training; unfortunately, you cannot assume that anyone advertising vasectomy reversals is truly prepared to give you the best procedure possible. With an investment of this magnitude—which, for most couples, is emotional as well as financial—I want you to have the knowledge you need to find a surgeon who can maximize your odds of success.

Vasectomy Reversal Cost

The average cost for a microsurgical vasectomy reversal performed by a urologist in the United States is around $10,000, although this can vary significantly depending on the region in which you live (New York City is generally going to be more expensive than Des Moines, Iowa, for example). When seeking a reversal specialist, you should be able to find out what the price will be by contacting the doctor's office (if it is not listed on a website). Be sure to ask about any additional costs beyond the surgeon's fee. Sometimes financing options may be available. High-volume reversal specialists are often able to negotiate lower facility fee prices with a surgery center, resulting in lower overall prices. For example, the total cost for a vasectomy reversal at my facility in southwest Ohio is currently around $6,300 (this is the total combined cost, including the procedure, anesthesia, and facility).

Optional Sperm Freezing

At the time of a vasectomy reversal, sperm can be frozen and stored as backup for IVF in case the reversal procedure is not successful. Sperm can be obtained from the vas deferens or directly from the testicle. My preference is to harvest testicular sperm, since these are fresh, newly made sperm, as opposed to the potentially old, stagnant sperm found in the vas deferens. Costs vary, but there is generally an additional charge for the extra surgery center time as well as a charge from the fertility lab for processing and freezing the sperm. In my practice, I personally do not charge more for extracting testicular sperm at the time of a reversal. The extra anesthesia and surgery center time costs $350, and the local fertility lab charges about $800 to process and freeze the sperm. The storage fee for sperm is generally around $275 per year.

Appendix A

Finding a Male Fertility Specialist

Identifying a urologist who specializes in male infertility can sometimes be challenging. General urology training programs do not place much emphasis on male fertility problems, with the result that the majority of urologists are not familiar with the latest guidelines and techniques for managing male infertility. Some urologists choose to pursue advanced fellowship training in male infertility management (andrology), and most large metropolitan areas have at least one urologist who is fellowship-trained in male infertility. Patients who live in smaller communities may need to either travel to a larger nearby city to find a male fertility specialist or find a general urologist who has decided to learn more about the management of male fertility problems.

A good online resource for finding a urologist who focuses on male infertility is the website of the Society for the Study of Male Reproduction (www.ssmr.org). This website has a "Find a Doctor" link that allows a search by geographic location. The SSMR does not check the background of its members, so it is still important to do some basic research to make sure that the doctor you are planning on seeing has the proper training and qualifications. Ideally this would include advanced fellowship training in andrology/male infertility, which can be verified by calling the urologists office.

For couples who cannot find a nearby male fertility specialist, one option is to call a local IVF practice and see which urologist they refer their male patients to. If there is no nearby IVF practice, then try local ob-gyn practices; they often know which nearby urologists specialize in male fertility.

Appendix B

Male Infertility Textbooks

The following are comprehensive textbooks on male infertility written for medical professionals:

Male Infertility: Contemporary Clinical Approaches, Andrology, ART & Antioxidants, by Sijo J. Parekattil and Ashok Agarwal (Springer, 2012)

Surgical and Medical Management of Male Infertility, by Marc Goldstein and Peter N. Schlegel (Cambridge University Press, 2013)

Infertility in the Male, by Larry I. Lipshultz, Stuart S. Howards, and Craig S. Niederberger (Cambridge University Press, 2009)

Appendix C

Fertility Evaluation and Treatment Pricing List

Lab Testing Costs

Table 1 below lists examples of laboratory test costs if you do not have insurance coverage. Coverage for infertility testing varies greatly from state to state, as well as between individual policies. Check with your insurance company to see if fertility testing will be covered. If not, I recommended that you do some research to find the lowest "cash pay" prices are in your area, since you can see from Table 1 that there is quite a range of prices for the same test.

The prices listed in Table 1 were obtained via phone calls to the laboratories in December 2014 and may have changed since that time, so always check to verify current pricing. The table includes a local lab from southwest Ohio (TriHealth) as well as two national laboratory companies (Quest and LabCorp). Companies such as LabCorp often have contracts with particular medical practices and offer the patients of these practices special rates on testing, so I've broken this down into two categories: "LabCorp" lists the general prices for anyone using a LabCorp facility, and "LabCorp with a contracted office" shows the rates when patients from a local medical practice that has contracted with LabCorp have the same testing. Integrated Genetics is a national genetics testing lab, and

Reprosource is a specialized company focusing on fertility-related lab tests.

Table 1: Lab Testing Costs

	Total T	Free T	Total T + free T/bioavailable T	FSH	LH	Estradiol
TriHealth	$89.60	$112.00	$173.99	$81.73	$81.47	$122.91
Quest/Compunet	$276.60	$522.23	$647.56	$196.74	$279.01	$326.70
LabCorp	$155.00	$199.00	$378.00	$107.00	$104.00	$174.00
LabCorp with contracted office	$14.00		$26.00	$19.00	$17.00	$20.00
Integrated Genetics (formerly Genzyme)						
Reprosource*	$85.00	$85.00		$55.00		$40.00

	Prolactin	Inhibin B	Karyotype	YCMD	Cystic fibrosis
TriHealth	$85.25	$245.00	$900.00	$813.00	$226.00 (97m + 5T)
Quest/Compunet	$227.13	$195.32	$1,690.69	$632.76	
LabCorp	$133.00	$294.00	$809.00	$354.00	$800.00 (97m), $1,055.00 (97m + 5T)
LabCorp with contracted office	$20.00		$338.00	$350.00	$200.00 (32m)
Integrated Genetics (formerly Genzyme)			$1134.00	$1229.00	$800.00 (97m), $309.00 (poly T)
Reprosource*	$43.00	$45.00	$487.00	$206.00	$380.00 (97m + 5T)

* Reprosource charges $50 for third-party mobile phlebotomy if not drawn at contracted lab. It also offers a hormone panel for $248.00 that includes testosterone (total, free, and bioavailable), FSH, LH, estradiol, inhibin B, and prolactin.

Sperm DNA testing is less widely available. Reprosource offers it for 175.00 +75.00 shipping, while SCSA Diagnostics offers it for 225.00 + 150.00 shipping.

Note to laboratory companies: if you have any updated information or corrections on the costs of your testing, or if you would like to add your company to this list for next year's edition, please email 10weekmanplan@gmail.com.

Fertility Medication Costs

There is a huge range of variability in the cost of fertility medications from pharmacy to pharmacy. As with the lab test pricing above, if you have insurance coverage for your fertility medications, then the choice of which pharmacy you are going to use is less important. However, many couples in the United States do not have insurance that covers fertility medications, so shopping around to find the best price can potentially save you quite a bit of money. Ask for the generic version of the medication when possible, as the pricing can vary dramatically (for example, at one point in time a month's supply of Clomid at Sam's Club costs $242.27, as compared with $24.00 for generic clomiphene at the same location).

Listed below are drug medication prices from December 2014, as obtained by phone calls to the pharmacies. These prices can change, so it is important to always verify the costs of these medications before you commit to purchasing them from a particular pharmacy. The Costco, Sam's Club, Walmart, Walgreens, and Kroger pharmacy pricing is from local stores in southwest Ohio, and prices may vary by region. The others are national pharmacies based in the United States that carry specialty fertility medications.

Table 2 lists the prices for clomiphene, anastrazole, and the three HCG formulations (generic HCG, Novarel, and Pregnyl). HCG prices are for a vial of 10,000 IU, and in brackets is the monthly cost if HCG is used at the standard starting dosage of

2,000 IU three times a week. "N/A" indicates that a pharmacy does not carry that particular medication as of December 2014.

Table 2: Costs for Clomiphene, Anastrazole, HCG

	Clomiphene 25 mg qd, 1-month supply	Anastrazole 1 mg qd, 1-month supply*
Costco	$23.75	$23.46 ($17.27 online)
Sam's Club	$24.00	$88.05
Walmart	$24.00	$109.22
Kroger	$24.00	$329.09
Walgreens	$51.99	$204.99
Walgreens Specialty Pharmacy*	$110.25	$495.00
Freedom Fertility	$55.35	$404.85
Apothecary by Design	$27.00	$739.11
Kings Fertility Pharmacy	$60.00	$30.00
Success Meds	$30.00	N/A
Barron Pharmacy	$117.00	$36.00

	Generic HCG, 10,000 IU vial [monthly cost]	Novarel, 10,000 IU vial [monthly cost]	Pregnyl, 10,000 IU vial [monthly cost]
Costco	N/A	$217.93 [$523.03]	$96.54 [$231.70]
Sam's Club	$284.57 [$682.97]	N/A	$80.70 [$193.68]
Walmart	N/A	$394.28 [$946.27]	$84.04 [$201.70]
Kroger	N/A	$254.79 [$611.50]	$101.89 [$244.54]
Walgreens	N/A	$241.99 [$580.78]	$112.99 [$271.18]
Walgreens Specialty Pharmacy*	$164.95 [$395.88]	$87.95 [$211.08]**	$92.00 [$220.80]
Freedom Fertility	$109.90 [$263.76]	$109.90 [$263.76]	$139.88 [$335.71]
Apothecary by Design	N/A	$88.00 [$211.20]	$86.00 [$206.40]
Kings Fertility Pharmacy	N/A	$89.99 [$215.98]	$89.99 [$215.98]
Success Meds	N/A	$109.00 [$261.60]	$99.99 [$239.98]
Barron Pharmacy	N/A	$99.75 [$239.40]	$82.68 [$198.43]

* Another option for anastrazole: If you do not have insurance coverage, you can mail an original prescription to Empower Pharmacy for $50.10 per month (for 1 mg daily dosage); the address is 12123 Jones Rd., Houston, TX 77070, 877-562-8577, www.EmpowerRx.Pharmacy.com. This is a compounding pharmacy that makes its own medications and is used by some fertility experts around the country.

** Walgreens Specialty Pharmacy offers discounted rates on some of its medications if you sign up for its discount program.

For online training in how to inject HCG, see www.freedomfertility.com, under "Injection Training for Infertility."

Table 3 lists the prices for cabergoline as well as four injectable FSH formulations. Standard dosage for FSH injections is 75 IU three times a week. Follistim comes in a 300 IU pre-loaded "pen," but there is actually more than 300 IU in each pen, so five injections of 75 IU can be given with each pen. Gonal-F has a 300 IU pen that contains four injections of 75 IU each. Menopur and Bravelle come in 75 IU individual vials. Pricing for the Follistim and Gonal-F are for each 300 IU pen, and in brackets is the monthly cost when used at 75 IU three times a week. For the Menopur and Bravelle the listed prices are for each 75 IU vial, and in brackets is the monthly cost for 75 IU three times a week.

Table 3: Costs for Cabergoline and FSH

	Cabergoline 0.5 mg tabs, #8
Costco	$73.22
Sam's Club	$185.27
Walmart	$211.52
Kroger	$230.09
Walgreens	$371.99
Walgreens Specialty Pharmacy*	$317.28
Freedom Fertility	$216.00
Apothecary by Design	$110.00
Kings Fertility Pharmacy	$130.00
Success Meds	$126.00
Barron Pharmacy	$186.00

	Follistim pen, 300 IU [monthly cost]	Gonal-F pen, 300 IU [monthly cost]	Menopur, 75 IU vial [monthly cost]	Bravelle, 75 IU vial [monthly cost]
Costco	$588.39 [$1,412.36]	$496.39 [$1,489.17]	N/A	$144.26 [$1,731.12]
Sam's Club	N/A	$636.05 [$1,908.15]	$141.18 [$1,694.16]	$125.50 [$1,506.00]
Walmart	$618.37 [$1,488.37]	$676.33 [$2,028.99]	$145.84 [$1,750.88]	$129.14 [$1,549.68]
Kroger	$679.39 [$1,630.54]	$637.29 [$1,911.87]	$164.49 [$1,973.88]	$148.99 [$1787.88]
Walgreens	N/A	$632.99 [$1,898.97]	$189.69 [$2,276.28]	$143.69 [$1,724.28]
Walgreens Specialty Pharmacy*	$268.00 [$643.20]*	$559.17 [$1,677.51]	$75.50 [$906.00]*	$60.66 [$727.92]*
Freedom Fertility	$639.60 [$1,535.04]	$304.00 [$912.00]	$68.90 [$826.80]	$62.90 [$754.80]
Apothecary by Design	$286.00 [$686.40]	$304.00 [$912.00]	$79.90 [$958.80]	$64.00 [$768.00]
Kings Fertility Pharmacy	$509.00 [$1,221.60]	$304.00 [$912.00]	$77.00 [$924.00]	$60.00 [$720.00]
Success Meds	$289.90 [$695.76]	N/A	$80.99 [$971.88]	$65.99 [$791.88]
Barron Pharmacy	$294.60 [$707.04]	$304.00 [$912.00]	$79.00 [$948.00]	$63.50 [$762.00]

* Walgreens Specialty Pharmacy offers discounted rates on some of its medications if you sign up for its discount program.

For online training in how to inject FSH, see www.freedomfertility.com, under "Injection Training for Infertility."

If you do not have insurance for these medications, look for a pharmacy with prices cheaper than those listed above. I recommend only using U.S.-based pharmacies, as the quality of medications produced outside of the United States cannot be verified, given lack of FDA supervision. If you find a cheaper place to purchase these medications, please let us know by emailing 10weekmanplan@gmail.com. I will then include the listing in next year's edition of this book, and you can help other couples to save money.

Note to pharmacies: If you have any updated information or corrections on the costs of your medications, or if you would like to add your pharmacy to the list for next year's edition, please email 10weekmanplan@gmail.com.

Appendix D

Fertility Treatment Options for Women

There is a wide variety of female fertility treatment options available; here I'll only briefly describe them. There are many good online and print resources on female fertility you can consult, an example of which is the book "The Fast Track to Fertility". Consulting with a specialist in female fertility is also an excellent source of information as well.

General Success Rates and Likelihood of Multiple Births

	Pregnancy rate per cycle	Likelihood of multiple births
Timed intercourse (after one year of trying)	3–5%	1%
Clomiphene plus timed intercourse	8–10%	10%
Intrauterine insemination (IUI), combined with clomiphene	15–20%	10%
In vitro fertilization (IVF)	35–45%	30%

The above chart shows approximate rates of pregnancy and the chance of multiple births for different treatments. These are general numbers; your specialist can provide you with more individualized estimated success rates that take into consideration your particular circumstances.

Medications

Hormonal medications such as clomiphene, tamoxifen, letrozole, and anastrazole are often effective in treating ovulatory dysfunction, with the goal of reestablishing normal ovulation. In women with otherwise normal ovulation, these medications can (modestly) increase the chance of pregnancy by producing a higher number of eggs than normal. This type of medication is generally taken for about five days, starting between day 3 and day 5 of the woman's cycle. They are inexpensive (generally costing under $50 per cycle), but do increase the risk of multiple births (up to 10 percent chance of twins, with less than 1 percent chance of triplets or other higher-order pregnancies). For the best chances of success, a total motile sperm count of at least 20 million is desirable when using natural intercourse combined with medications, though men with lower total motile counts may be successful as well.

General ob-gyns often feel comfortable prescribing medications like clomiphene. If three or four cycles of these medications do not result in pregnancy, the chance of success with additional cycles starts to decrease significantly, and women are typically encouraged to think about moving on to other treatment options, such as intrauterine insemination.

Intrauterine Insemination

Also known as artificial insemination, intrauterine insemination (IUI) involves placing the man's sperm directly into his partner's uterus at the correct time during her ovulatory cycle. A woman undergoing IUI is often given medications such as clomiphene, although natural-cycle IUI can be performed without any medications. The addition of medications can increase the chances of success modestly, but it also increases the risk of multiple births (to about 10 percent).

The woman is generally monitored by blood tests or intravaginal ultrasound, and at the time of her peak fertility, just before ovulation, the man is asked to give a semen sample. The sperm are processed (washed and concentrated) and placed into the woman's uterus through a slender tube; this is typically not much more painful than a Pap smear.

A minimum of 5 million pre-wash total motile sperm or 1 million post-wash total motile sperm is needed for a decent chance of success; higher total motile sperm counts do increase the chances of pregnancy. Sometimes double collections are performed to increase the number of sperm that are inseminated. Some reproductive endocrinologists recommend natural intercourse either right before or right after an IUI as well. Pooling of multiple frozen semen specimens for IUI can be performed, but in general 50 to 75 percent of the sperm from each sample do not survive the freeze/thaw process, so fresh specimens are best when they are available.

Some general ob-gyns perform IUI in their office. However, most ob-gyns prefer to refer women to a fertility specialist for insemination.

The cost for IUI ranges between $400 and $1,600 for each cycle.

Intrauterine Insemination with Gonadotropins

IUI can be combined with the use of gonadotropins by the woman in order to generate a larger number of eggs. This is associated with higher pregnancy rates, but the trade-off is increased cost—the hormonal medications can be expensive. The risk of multiple births is also higher. The chance of higher-order births (triplets or more) is greatest when IUI is combined with gonadotropins, since there is no control over the number of eggs that are released and potentially fertilized within the woman's reproductive tract.

In Vitro Fertilization

Standard in vitro fertilization (IVF) involves extracting eggs from the woman and mixing them directly with sperm in the lab. A variant of this, called intracytoplasmic sperm injection (ICSI), involves injecting a single sperm into each egg. Fewer sperm are required for ICSI, making it the procedure of choice for men who can only produce small numbers of sperm. ICSI can also bypass problems with egg/sperm interactions, and is recommended for men with very low strict morphology readings (under 3–4%) and for couples who have had multiple failures with standard IVF for unknown reasons. In both standard IVF and ICSI, the woman is injected with medications that increase the number of eggs she produces in each cycle. The eggs are removed under transvaginal ultrasound guidance and combined with the sperm. After the fertilized eggs (now called embryos) have been allowed to mature for a few days, two to four embryos (depending on factors such as the woman's age, the quality of the embryos, etc.) are transferred into the woman's uterus. Any remaining embryos can be frozen for later use.

IVF protocols are constantly being modified to improve outcomes. Current trends include the transfer of only one embryo (called single embryo transfer). Already common in Europe, this practice has the potential to dramatically decrease the number of higher-order pregnancies, but it has the trade-off of a potentially lower pregnancy rate per cycle. Other current trends include freezing all embryos and then transferring them to the woman later, when the uterus has returned to a more normal physiologic environment (as opposed to the hyperstimulated state that a fresh embryo is transferred into); potential benefits in terms of pregnancy outcomes as well as the future health implications for the embryo and baby are being investigated.

There are a number of common concerns associated with IVF:

- *Cost.* IVF is expensive, with a typical cycle costing between $10,000 and $15,000.

- *Increased risk of birth defects.* The vast majority of babies born to couples undergoing IVF are normal, but there is some evidence that rates of rare birth defects are higher than in natural pregnancies. It is unclear whether this slightly elevated risk is due to changes in the woman's hormonal environment, loss of the egg's natural selection process of excluding defective sperm (with ICSI), or some other factor.

- *What to do with unused frozen embryos.* Several options exist, including embryo donation.

- *Hyperstimulation.* A small number of women create too many eggs during the stimulation phase, which can lead to potentially serious complications and hospitalization.

Your female fertility specialist can provide you with more information about each of these concerns, as well as strategies to navigate these potential problems.

Data for National IVF Outcomes, 2012

	Age of woman				
	< 35	35–37	38–40 years	41–42 years	> 42
Pregnancy rate	46.7%	37.8%	29.7%	19.8%	8.6%
Live birth rate	40.7%	31.3%	22.2%	11.8%	3.9%
Twins	29.5%	25.0%	20.3%	13.4%	9.0%
Triplets or more	1.1%	0.7%	0.7%	0.7%	0.4%
Live birth rate, frozen embryo transfer	42.4%	39.8%	33.9%	26.4%	17.8%
Live birth rate, fresh transfer	47.1%	37.9%	28.5%	16.3%	6.1%
Live birth rate, elective single embryo transfer	14.8%	8.9%	3.0%	1.2%	0.6%

Source: Society for Assisted Reproductive Technologies

The Society for Assisted Reproductive Technologies (SART) is a national professional organization that provides information to both patients and medical providers regarding the IVF process. SART also reports IVF outcomes for almost all of the IVF programs in the United States, with a lag time of several years (to accumulate and process the data). The chart above shows the latest IVF outcomes for which data are available (2012) for all U.S. IVF programs. The SART website (www.sart.org) contains a map listing the IVF programs in each state, as well as the statistics of that program's IVF outcomes based upon a number of factors, including the woman's age.

Typical IVF Cycle

Here's how a typical cycle of IVF works:

1. The woman takes an oral contraceptive for fourteen to twenty-one days, starting on day 4 of her menstrual cycle. This reduces the chance of hyperstimulation and ovarian cyst formation. Women who have decreased ovarian reserve usually skip this step.

2. A GnRH agonist (such as Lupron) is taken for twelve to fifteen days. This temporarily shuts down the ovaries, preventing premature ovulation and ensuring that all of the eggs for this cycle mature at the same time.

3. A gonadotropin (e.g., Gonal F) is administered for ten to twelve days, to stimulate ovarian egg production. During this period the woman is monitored regularly with ultrasound and blood tests.

4. An injection of human chorionic gonadotropin (HCG) is given, to cause final maturation of the eggs.

5. The eggs are retrieved, generally around thirty-six hours after the HCG injection.

6. The eggs are fertilized in the lab and allowed to mature for three to five days.

7. The embryos are transferred to the woman's uterus, and progesterone is administered to support implantation.

8. A pregnancy test is done fourteen days after retrieval or transfer.

9. If pregnancy results, two ultrasounds are done: the first either two weeks after a positive pregnancy test or at 6.5–7.5 weeks of pregnancy, and the second at 7.5–8.5 weeks of pregnancy.

10. After 8 to 10 weeks of pregnancy, the woman's care is transferred from the specialist back to her regular ob-gyn for the remainder of the pregnancy.

This is only a rough guide; your particular IVF cycle may proceed somewhat differently, based on your fertility specialist's preference, the particular clinical situation, and how the cycle is progressing.

IVF Terminology (by Day of Cycle)

Day 0:	Egg retrieval
Day 1:	Fertilization
Day 2:	Cleavage to 2-cell stage
Day 3:	8-cell stage
Day 4:	Morula stage (around 30 cells)
Day 5:	Blastocyst stage (generally 50–150 cells)

Appendix E

Osteoporosis

Many different factors can impact men's bone health, including hormones, diet, exercise, and genetics. From a hormonal standpoint, adequate testosterone and estradiol levels are important for maintaining good bone strength. Low testosterone and estradiol levels are known risk factors for the weakening of bones in men, making them more susceptible to fractures as they age.

Bone strength (also called bone mineral density, or BMD) is significantly influenced by:

- Hypogonadism (low testosterone)
- Nutrition
- Lifestyle (including tobacco use, alcohol use, and exercise)
- Medications (such as glucocorticoid steroids)
- Chronic disease
- Heredity

Bone density is usually measured by dual energy X-ray absorptiometry (DEXA) scanning. This is a quick X-ray of the hip and spine that directly measures bone density. A T-score is then given that compares that patient's peak bone density with normal values for his age, sex, and race. *Osteoporosis* is typically defined as having a T-score of -2.5 or lower (2.5 standard deviations or more below the mean), and it puts men at a greater risk for developing a fracture, especially in the spine, proximal femur (hip), and distal radius (wrist). *Osteopenia,* a lesser degree of bone weakening, is usually defined as having a T-score between -1.0 and -2.5.

Men who have a low total testosterone (less than 300 ng/dL) are generally advised to follow osteoporosis prevention guidelines in order to prevent worsening of bone mineral density. Some clinicians suggest that men with a very low total testosterone (less than 200 ng/dL) have a baseline DEXA scan to see if osteoporosis or osteopenia is already present. If the DEXA scan is abnormal, then it should be repeated in two years to see if the recommended interventions have been effective.

General guidelines for the prevention of osteoporosis and osteopenia:

- Calcium 1,000–1,500 mg daily
- Vitamin D 800 IU daily
- Regular weight-bearing exercise: three to five sessions (20 to 25 minutes each) each week of exercise such as jogging or running, skiing, weightlifting, or most ball sports
- Weight loss if overweight or obese (to bring BMI down to under 25)
- Avoid tobacco products and excessive alcohol intake
- Correction of low testosterone levels

If these measures are not effective in reversing osteoporotic/osteopenic changes, then stronger medications (such as bisphosphonates) are available that can increase bone strength. Special diagnostic tests, such as the Fracture Risk Assessment (FRAX) tool, developed by the World Health Organization, can be utilized to see if these stronger medications may be clinically indicated. Bisphosphonates work by inhibiting the normal bodily process of bone breakdown; medications in this category come in both oral forms, including alendronate (Fosamax) and risendronate (Actonel), and intravenous forms, including zolendronic acid (Zometa) and pamidronate (Aredia).

Estradiol Levels and Osteoporosis

In addition to testosterone, adequate estradiol levels also play a very important role in maintaining bone strength in men. Most experts believe that for adequate bone health, men should try to maintain long-term estradiol levels of at least 20 pg/mL if possible. Some men taking aromatase inhibitors (such as anastrazole) can have estradiol levels that fall below this range. These men should follow the basic osteoporosis guidelines listed above, consider periodic DEXA scanning if on aromatase inhibitors for a prolonged time, and stop taking them when they are done with their fertility efforts.

Clomiphene and Osteoporosis

The relationship between clomiphene and osteoporosis is still unclear. On one hand, clomiphene can increase both testosterone and estradiol levels, which should enhance bone health. However, the variable impact of clomiphene on different sets of estrogen receptors throughout the body raises concerns as to whether this medication can actually worsen osteoporosis over time. Studies have shown conflicting results, with some showing improvements in bone density and others showing decreased bone density in men using clomiphene. Because of these concerns, men who are done with their fertility efforts should stop taking clomiphene. If they are taking the medication for a prolonged period of time, they should consider periodic DEXA scanning.

Appendix F

Using Donor Sperm

Some couples choose to use donor sperm when they find themselves in circumstances where the man does not have any sperm to use, he has sperm but it is ineffective in establishing a pregnancy, or the couple does not want to use the sperm because of possible genetic abnormalities. Although many couples initially feel reluctant to use donor sperm, most who eventually choose this route are quite satisfied with the outcome and have no later regrets.

Sperm can be donated by family members or friends, or can be obtained from commercial sperm banks. Donor sperm can be used with intrauterine insemination (IUI), intracervical insemination (IC), or natural insemination (via intercourse with the donor).

Commercial Sperm Bank Selection Process

A common misconception is that sperm donation is not a very selective process. In reality, most of the more than 150 commercial sperm banks in the United States accept less than 5 percent of men applying to be sperm donors, and sometimes less than 1 percent. About 50 to 90 percent of sperm donors are college students or graduate students, and most fulfill the following criteria:

1. 18–39 years old
2. Negative for infectious disease:

- No history of significant risk factors for infectious disease

- Sperm is quarantined for six months before it can be used

- Regular testing for, e.g., HIV, hepatitis, gonorrhea, chlamydia, syphilis, cytomegalovirus

3. Genetic testing and full multigenerational family history to screen for diseases

4. No history of:
   - Blood transfusions within the last year
   - Homosexual activity
   - IV drug use
   - Genital herpes

5. Minimum quality of sperm:
   - Semen analysis of frozen/thawed sperm shows a minimum post-thaw density of 20×10^6 motile sperm/cc, 25–40 percent motility
   - Must maintain minimum sperm quality parameters for six months

6. Willing to provide two specimens a week

I recommend that you request and carefully review the screening criteria used by the specific commercial sperm bank that you are considering using.

Choosing a Commercial Sperm Donor

A wide range of criteria can be used by couples to select a donor who resembles the prospective father, if so desired. These criteria can include age, height, weight, eye and hair color, education, occupation, ethnicity, and religion. Donors can also be selected with the help of face-matching software that compares donor photos to a photo of the prospective father.

Tracking by Commercial Sperm Banks

Commercial sperm banks are required to keep track of any children who are born with birth defects or mental deficiencies (the average risk in the general population is 3–4 percent, and thus this should be the approximate risk in the donor population as well, minus any genetic issues that have been screened for). Most countries limit the number of children that can be born per donor (generally around ten) to decrease the risk of consanguinity later in life (having children with someone closely genetically related to you). Usually a donor who has reached his limit can provide further samples if a couple wants more sperm to try for additional biologically related siblings.

Sperm are usually donated in an anonymous fashion, in which the children do not have later access to the contact information of the sperm donor. Some labs do offer an "ID option," in which the donors agree that their offspring can contact them once the children reach eighteen years of age.

Cost of Donor Sperm

In general, using donor sperm costs around $500 per cycle. Listed below are the 2014 prices for three national sperm banks.

	Fairfax Cryobank	California Cryobank	Cryogenics Lab
ICI (unwashed 10 million TMC/cc)			
Anonymous	$498	$550	$380
ID option	$619	$650	$497
IUI (pre-washed 10 million TMC/cc)			
Anonymous	$625	$650	$450
ID option	$738	$750	$610
IVF (unwashed 5 million TM/cc)			
Anonymous	$360	NA	$250
ID option	$479	NA	$359

Appendix G

My Semen Analysis Parameters

Use this chart to fill in your personal semen analysis parameters. As you read "How to Interpret the Results of Semen Analysis" in Chapter 3, you can use this chart as a reference to see how your parameters match up with what is considered normal. If you have had more than three semen analysis tests, use the three most recent ones.

Semen Analysis Review	Test #1 Date: __/__/__	Test #2 Date: __/__/__	Test #3 Date: __/__/__	Normal Range
Volume of ejaculate				1.0 cc or more
Sperm density				20×10^6/cc (20 million sperm per cc) or more
Sperm motility				50% or more
Grade of motility				Grade 2 or higher
Sperm morphology				Greater than 4% by Kruger strict criteria or greater than 29% by WHO criteria
Total motile sperm count (Volume × density × percent motility)				40×10^6 (40 million sperm) or more
Semen pH (not always performed)				Higher than 7.4
Fructose (not always performed)				Positive
Viscosity/liquefaction				Viscosity 2 or less, or liquefaction in 30 minutes or less
White blood cells				1×10^6/cc or less (or under 10–15/hpf)
Clumping of sperm (typically reported in comments section if present)				No clumping (if present, may be consistent with the presence of anti-sperm antibodies)

Appendix H

Personal Fertility Profile

Section 1

Abnormal Semen Analysis Factors (from Appendix D)	Circle One	If Yes, See This Section
Low ejaculate volume (< 1.0 cc)	No / Yes	Chapter 6, "Reversible Semen Parameter Factors"
Acidic semen pH (< 7.5) or fructose negative	No / Yes	Chapter 6, "Reversible Semen Parameter Factors"
Abnormal viscosity or liquefaction (viscosity > 2 or liquefaction > 30 minutes)	No / Yes	Chapter 6, "Reversible Semen Parameter Factors"
Pyospermia (WBCs > 1 × 10^6/cc, or > 15/hpf)	No / Yes	Chapter 6, "Reversible Semen Parameter Factors"
Clumping of sperm present with low motility	No / Yes	Chapter 6, "Reversible Semen Parameter Factors"

Section 2

Demographics	Circle One	If Yes, See This Section
Age 45 or older	No / Yes	Chapter 6, "Demographic Factors That Can Impact Male Fertility"
Overweight (body mass index > 25)*	No / Yes	Chapter 6, "Demographic Factors That Can Impact Male Fertility"
Underweight (body mass index < 20)*	No / Yes	Chapter 6, "Demographic Factors That Can Impact Male Fertility"

Online calculators available, or use this formula:

$$\frac{\text{Weight in pounds} \times 703}{(\text{Height in inches})^2}$$

Section 3

Lifestyle	Circle One	If Yes, See This Section
Smoke cigarettes	No / Yes	Chapter 6, "Lifestyle-Related Fertility Issues"
Use smokeless tobacco	No / Yes	Chapter 6, "Lifestyle-Related Fertility Issues"
Use illicit drugs (marijuana, cocaine, etc.)	No / Yes	Chapter 6, "Lifestyle-Related Fertility Issues"
Drink more than 4 alcoholic drinks per week	No / Yes	Chapter 6, "Lifestyle-Related Fertility Issues"
Use hot tubs/saunas sometimes	No / Yes	Chapter 6, "Lifestyle-Related Fertility Issues"
Use a laptop computer directly on your lap sometimes	No / Yes	Chapter 6, "Lifestyle-Related Fertility Issues"
Take hot showers and/or baths	No / Yes	Chapter 6, "Lifestyle-Related Fertility Issues"
Use a seat warmer in the car	No / Yes	Chapter 6, "Lifestyle-Related Fertility Issues"
Wear tight underpants	No / Yes	Chapter 6, "Lifestyle-Related Fertility Issues"
Carry a cell phone in your pocket or on your belt	No / Yes	Chapter 6, "Lifestyle-Related Fertility Issues"
Use a cell phone more than 4 hours per day	No / Yes	Chapter 6, "Lifestyle-Related Fertility Issues"
Use lubricants during intercourse	No / Yes	Chapter 6, "Lifestyle-Related Fertility Issues"
Drink caffeinated coffee, tea, cola, or energy drinks	No / Yes	Chapter 6, "Lifestyle-Related Fertility Issues"
Exercise less than 30 minutes 3–4 days a week	No / Yes	Chapter 6, "Lifestyle-Related Fertility Issues"
Ride a bike more than 25 miles per week	No / Yes	Chapter 6, "Lifestyle-Related Fertility Issues"
Eat soy products on a regular basis	No / Yes	Chapter 6, "Lifestyle-Related Fertility Issues"

Section 4

Job-Related Issues	Circle One	If Yes, See This Section
Sit for prolonged periods of time	No / Yes	Chapter 6, "Job-Related Factors"
Have significant heat exposure	No / Yes	Chapter 6, "Job-Related Factors"
Feel like you are under a lot of stress	No / Yes	Chapter 6, "Job-Related Factors"
Have exposure to toxins and/or chemicals	No / Yes	Chapter 6, "Job-Related Factors"
Have exposure to significant amounts of air pollution	No / Yes	Chapter 6, "Job-Related Factors"

Section 5

Medications and Supplements	Circle One	If Yes, See This Section
Take prescription medications	No / Yes	Chapter 6, "Medications and Supplements"
Take non-prescription supplements	No / Yes	Chapter 6, "Medications and Supplements"
Take hormonally active substances (testosterone, DHEA, anabolic steroids, prohormones, T boosters)	No / Yes	Chapter 6, "Exogenous Androgens"

Section 6

History of Any of the Following Conditions	Circle One	If Yes, See This Section
Androgen insensitivity syndrome	No / Yes	Chapter 6, "Glossary of Fertility-Related Medical Problems"
Beta thalassemia	No / Yes	Chapter 6, "Glossary of Fertility-Related Medical Problems"
Celiac disease	No / Yes	Chapter 6, "Glossary of Fertility-Related Medical Problems"
Ciliary diseases (Kartagener's syndrome, immotile cilia syndrome)	No / Yes	Chapter 6, "Glossary of Fertility-Related Medical Problems"

Cirrhosis, liver disease	No / Yes	Chapter 6, "Glossary of Fertility-Related Medical Problems"
Congenital adrenal hyperplasia	No / Yes	Chapter 6, "Glossary of Fertility-Related Medical Problems"
Crohn's disease	No / Yes	Chapter 6, "Glossary of Fertility-Related Medical Problems"
Cryptorchidism (undescended testicles)	No / Yes	Chapter 6, "Glossary of Fertility-Related Medical Problems"
Chemotherapy or radiation therapy	No / Yes	Chapter 6, "Glossary of Fertility-Related Medical Problems"
Diabetes	No / Yes	Chapter 6, "Glossary of Fertility-Related Medical Problems"
Epididymitis	No / Yes	Chapter 6, "Glossary of Fertility-Related Medical Problems"
Glucocorticoid excess, Cushing's disease	No / Yes	Chapter 6, "Glossary of Fertility-Related Medical Problems"
Hemochromatosis	No / Yes	Chapter 6, "Glossary of Fertility-Related Medical Problems"
Hypospadias	No / Yes	Chapter 6, "Glossary of Fertility-Related Medical Problems"
Inguinal hernia repair	No / Yes	Chapter 6, "Glossary of Fertility-Related Medical Problems"
Myelodysplasia or spina bifida	No / Yes	Chapter 6, "Glossary of Fertility-Related Medical Problems"
Myotonic dystrophy	No / Yes	Chapter 6, "Glossary of Fertility-Related Medical Problems"
Orchitis or mumps	No / Yes	Chapter 6, "Glossary of Fertility-Related Medical Problems"
Pituitary insufficiency (hypopituitarism)	No / Yes	Chapter 6, "Glossary of Fertility-Related Medical Problems"
Polycystic kidney disease	No / Yes	Chapter 6, "Glossary of Fertility-Related Medical Problems"
Posterior urethral valves	No / Yes	Chapter 6, "Glossary of Fertility-Related Medical Problems"
Prader-Willi syndrome	No / Yes	Chapter 6, "Glossary of Fertility-Related Medical Problems"
Prostatitis	No / Yes	Chapter 6, "Glossary of Fertility-Related Medical Problems"
Prune belly syndrome	No / Yes	Chapter 6, "Glossary of Fertility-Related Medical Problems"
Renal failure	No / Yes	Chapter 6, "Glossary of Fertility-

		Related Medical Problems"
Retractile testicles	No / Yes	Chapter 6, "Glossary of Fertility-Related Medical Problems"
Sarcoidosis	No / Yes	Chapter 6, "Glossary of Fertility-Related Medical Problems"
Sickle cell anemia	No / Yes	Chapter 6, "Glossary of Fertility-Related Medical Problems"
Spinal cord injury or disease	No / Yes	Chapter 6, "Glossary of Fertility-Related Medical Problems"
Testicular cancer	No / Yes	Chapter 6, "Glossary of Fertility-Related Medical Problems"
Testicular torsion	No / Yes	Chapter 6, "Glossary of Fertility-Related Medical Problems"
Urethral stricture disease	No / Yes	Chapter 6, "Glossary of Fertility-Related Medical Problems"
Young's syndrome	No / Yes	Chapter 6, "Glossary of Fertility-Related Medical Problems"

Section 7

Sexual History	Circle One	If Yes, See This Section
Problems with erections	No / Yes	Chapter 6, "Erectile Dysfunction"
Problems with ejaculation	No / Yes	Chapter 6, "Ejaculatory Problems"

Section 8

Varicocele	Circle One	If Yes, See This Section
Clinically significant varicocele by physical exam or ultrasound	No / Yes	Chapter 6, "Varicoceles"

Section 9

Review of Hormone Testing	Your Result	Normal Range	If Outside Normal Range, See This Section
Testosterone		< 500 ng/dL	Chapter 7
Bioavailable testosterone		< 156 ng/dL	Chapter 7
Free testosterone		< 15 ng/dL (direct) < 50 ng/dL (calculated)	Chapter 7
Estradiol		≥ 59mg/mL	Chapter 7
Testosterone-to-estradiol (T/E) ratio		< 10:1	Chapter 7
FSH		1.0–7.0 IU/L	Chapter 7
TSH		0.4–3.0 µIU/mL	Chapter 7
Prolactin		≥ 25 mcg/L	Chapter 7
, LH		1.0–8.0 IU/L	Chapter 7
Inhibin B		< 173 pg/mL	Chapter 7

Appendix I

Sample Semen Analysis Order Form

Date: ___/___/_____

Patient Name: _____

Date of Birth: ___/___/_____

<u>Semen Analysis Testing</u>

(Including Sperm Density, Motility, and Morphology)

Dx: V26.21

(Z31.41 after October 1, 2015)

3–4 days of abstinence prior to testing.

Please fax the results to: _____-_____-_____

Signed: _____

Provider Name:_____

Office Phone Number: _____-_____-_____

Appendix J

Sample Blood Test Order Form

Date: ___/___/_____

Patient Name: _____

Date of Birth: ___/___/_____

Blood Hormone Testing

Please draw all lab tests that are checked

☐ Total testosterone   (draw 7:00–10:00 a.m.)

☐ Bioavailable testosterone (draw 7:00–10:00 a.m.)

☐ Estradiol

☐ FSH

☐ LH

☐ Prolactin

☐ Other: _____

☐ Other: _____

Dx: 257.2

(E29.1 after October 1, 2015)

Please fax the results to: _____-_____-_____

Signed: _____

Provider Name: _____

Office Phone Number: _____-_____-_____

Appendix K

Scrotal Ultrasound Protocol

Give this form to the ultrasonographer before your evaluation.

The goal of this scrotal ultrasound is to evaluate for the presence of a clinically significant varicocele as well as any other scrotal abnormalities.

A clinically significant varicocele is defined as a dilated vein > 3.5 mm in the standing position that exhibits retrograde flow when a Valsalva procedure is performed. It is important to evaluate for varicoceles *with the patient in the standing position.*

Please record in your final report:

1. Testicular size
2. Presence of testicular masses
3. Any other scrotal findings (hydrocele, epididymal cysts, etc.)
4. Diameter of largest vein in the standing position
5. The presence of retrograde blood flow in the largest vein with Valsalva (in the standing position)
6. Any other noted abnormalities

Thank you for your assistance.

Appendix L

Transrectal Ultrasound Protocol

Give this form to the ultrasonographer before your evaluation.

The following aspects of the anatomy of the prostate, seminal vesicles and ejaculatory ducts are being evaluated to assess their potential impact on fertility.

1. Prostate

   a. Size

   b. Lesions/cysts: size, location (central, peripheral, etc.)

2. Seminal vesicles

   a. Maximal length (cm) for each side

   b. Maximal width (cm) for each side (normal max width 0.4–1.4 cm; abnormal max width >1.5cm)

   c. Presence of abnormalities (cysts, masses, air/fluid levels, etc.)

3. Ejaculatory duct

   a. Presence of dilation

   b. If dilated, maximal width (cm) (normal max width 0.04–0.08 cm; abnormal max width > 0.23 cm)

   c. Abnormalities along duct (stones, cysts, calcifications, etc.)

4. Any other standard TRUS findings noted

Thank you for your assistance.

54900035R00232

Made in the USA
Lexington, KY
02 September 2016

A Truly Comprehensive Guide for Couples with Male Factor Fertility Problems and Unexplained Infertility

The culmination of nearly a decade of clinical experience, this book is the first of its kind written by a fellowship-trained expert in male fertility. This step-by-step guide was designed for all couples experiencing male fertility issues or unexplained fertility problems, including:

- Couples just getting started (no male fertility testing yet)
- Men with abnormal semen analysis findings
- Normal semen analysis (and normal female testing) but still unable to conceive a child
- Men who are unable to successfully provide a specimen for semen analysis testing
- Recurrent pregnancy loss
- Recurrent IVF failure
- Previous vasectomy

The book was written to provide a framework for understanding the various possible causes of male fertility problems. Personalized questionnaires help couples to focus on the issues pertinent to their situation and efficiently lead them along the path from appropriate testing and diagnosis to effective management approaches. Advice on how to identify a skilled local medical provider is offered, as well as up-to-date comparative pricing information on fertility lab testing and commonly used medications.

Infertility is a common problem impacting millions of couples every year. The 10 Week Man Plan was written to provide couples with the knowledge and tools that they need to effectively and efficiently maximize their male fertility potential and help them to finally start a family of their own.

ISBN 9780986353222

90000 >

9 780986 353222